DARK SIDE
OF A
MOUNTAIN

VERONIKA VALDOVA

DEDICATION

The book is dedicated to all physicians and clinical research professionals who do the right thing for the right reasons.

TABLE OF CONTENTS

i

I. THE CODE

Medical profession has always been a special one. Unique social status of doctors stemmed from the power they had over people's lives, for their ability to heal the wounded and to bring the sick back to life; a status which was at times of hardship perceived as closer to God than to ordinary human beings. This noble profession requires many years of dedication to master the skills required to understand and uplift human body. The profession also requires an oath which goes back to the times of ancient Greece and which requires medical practitioners newly accepted into the ranks to treat their patients to their best knowledge and act in the interest of their patients. Some oaths also include a clause on physician's duty not to take into account the patient's social status. The uncomfortable truth that not all patients can afford the same level of care does inevitably come up; and in most societies both ancient and contemporary the poor receive some level of solidarity from those who are better off, although the extent of this solidarity can be very limited. Medical profession and priesthood, professions so close that they sometimes merged in one, compare to the keepers of gate to the underworld. People enter the world and leave it in the presence of medical professionals and priests, and expect them to provide assistance at times of crises.

THE BOOK OF LEVITICUS

Leviticus, the third book of the Bible, is divided into 27 chapters in which offerings to Lord for various sins are described; as well as ways how to treat those who are unclean, and how to make them clean again; how to preserve cleanliness of food; and how to maintain long-term health of their communities. Leviticus is probably the oldest written code of food hygiene, epidemiology, and reproduction and community health. This community health code imposed on the peoples of Israel contains many rules which are still relevant today. In historical context they certainly did have justification based on empirical experience and contemporary knowledge. The role of guardians of human health at population level did not belong to medical professionals though, but to the priests. Priest was the authority that had the power to pronounce a person or a house clean and unclean; and to impose remedies which would prevent spreading of a contagious disease to others. The code presents in great detail animals and foods which shall not be eaten by people, and sometimes not even touched to preserve cleanliness of an individual and the community. Leviticus, the third book of the Bible, prioritizes health and well-being of the community over the rights and well-being of an individual. Those who were unclean were openly ostracized, and only allowed to socialize when they became clean again; while those wicked and deformed, either physically or mentally, were excluded from society and from reproduction. From population perspective, higher death rate was compensated by higher birth rate. This directly relates to ban on methods limiting reproduction and ban on abortion. Social pathologies were then consistently punished by death. This is the original code which is still used by some Middle Eastern cultures to this day. There is very little difference between the teachings of Quran and the Old Testament, and it cannot be overlooked that they both stem from the same source. The only substantial difference is that the secular Euro-American civilization no longer considers these ancient teachings binding because it had the time and opportunity to evolve and develop a sophisticated parallel legal system which is, in the difference from religious teachings, binding for all members of society as defined by the respective jurisdiction, and not just for followers of a specific faith. Religion and legal system separated in two already under the Romans. In ancient Rome, monotheistic Jewish community was more or less allowed to govern itself by its own laws. The character of Jesus is portrayed in all four gospels in minute detail and with great consistency. In the absence of forensic evidence, books of the Bible are the only proof available with regards to physical existence of Jesus. The Romans reserved death by crucifixion for rebels against the Roman State. Crucifixion of Jesus is described in all four gospels in graphic detail, and is also mentioned in other historical records including Tacitus in parts where he elaborates on Pontius Pilate and Emperor Tiberius. Jesus, the King of the Jews, was perceived as political threat to the Roman State because of his subversive teachings. As per Harvey's book 'Jesus and the constraints of history'[1], early Christians denied any such activity and portrayed Jesus only as a religious teacher and not as a freedom fighter.

The legal grounds for his crucifixion remain rather obscure and historians still consider several possible scenarios. As mentioned by Philo of Alexandria, Pontius Pilate frequently carried out executions without trial and the possibility of crucifixion of an innocent person through miscarriage of justice or simple abuse of power cannot be ruled out. There is also the possibility that the verdict was influenced by pressure from the Jewish community itself and Jesus was executed to meet popular demand, simply because his teachings were very provocative, and because he attracted high degree of animosity among fellow Jews. Jesus's arrival to the Mount of Olives on a donkey was a monumental provocation since he had the authority to require transport. Excitement of the crowds did not last long though. He could have been handed over to the Romans after being condemned to death for blasphemy although this possibility is denied by Luke who clearly stated that Jesus was not found guilty by any Jewish court. Luke, Paul, and Peter sing in consonance that those who are found guilty of blasphemy and idolatry shall be put to death by 'hanging upon wood' (crucifixion). The reasons for him being handed over

---

[1] Harvey, AE. 1982. *Jesus and the Constraints of History*. Westminster John Knox Press.

to the Romans could be envy and jealousy as concluded by Mark or sheer ignorance which is what Luke apparently thought about the motivations.

Jesus's attitude to Jewish law was highly disrespectful and provocative, especially his violations of food laws and transgressions of Sabbath. True is that the violations were not prosecuted. Food laws are still central to Jewish religion today. Jesus pronounced all foods clean and human waste unclean, and did not fast. He did not wash his hands before meals and did not share the ambition of the Code of Conduct. Jesus provoked the community among other things by the company he kept because he rejected the traditional Jewish social exclusiveness. In essence, Jesus challenged Jewish way of life and by challenging the Law of Moses. Many perceived Jesus was a false prophet and believed that the name 'Christ' he used meant 'end of the Law'. Jesus demanded noting less but extension of the Laws of Moses from the 'Code of Conduct' or 'Change of Behavior' to much more profound transformation, and that was change in the 'Way of Thinking'. While Moses required people to refrain from 'homicide' and 'adultery', Jesus asked them to go much further and refrain from 'anger' which is the core emotion leading to homicide, and 'desire' which is the core cause of 'adultery'. The Laws of Moses pay lot of attention to damages in law and compensations for insult or injury. Jesus's demand was not only to refrain from insulting and harming others, but also to show love to one's enemies. It was Jesus who renounced the option of divorce which was present in Jewish law.

The moment in history was widely perceived as exceptional. The general excitement of the masses led to neglect of duties which would otherwise be intolerable, such as the tradition to bury one's own parents expressed as 'Let the dead bury their dead'. There was a widespread expectation of an imminent end, a kind of apocalypse, the end of history or a significant change, such as new social order. No matter how controversial figure Jesus was when he was alive, he was acknowledged as a prophet by all. The name 'Messiah' was understood by all without further description. No end of history occurred; but dis-confirmation of prophecy does not diminish credibility of a prophet. Jesus did not conform to a known pattern of a healer, magician, shaman, or exorcist; and was believed to possess extraordinary powers of prolonged concentration which is rather common among Buddhist monks. The diseases he cured were those which were disabling but curable using natural phenomena not widely known and understood at that time.

The choice of name became eventually the core of the claim. Calling himself 'Jesus the Christ' meant that he did lay a claim on his Messianic status. If Jesus was 'authorized' to act as he did which means as the Son of God, he must have been either obeyed and followed or eliminated for blasphemy. While Christians acknowledged his claim for Messianic status and followed his teachings, the Jews did not. The Christian doctrine in fact challenged the oneness of God but this was never understood by the Jews in literal sense of this claim, just like the virgin birth which is central to Christianity.

But this is not the only possible explanation of the reasons of his crucifixion. There is also a possibility that Jesus offered himself to the authorities as a ransom for many to prevent genocide of the entire nation. This explanation was offered by Caiaphus who advised Sandherin that Jesus shall be handed over to the Romans to be executed rather than the whole race to be destroyed. In this sense this would be a reminiscence of the attempted genocide and the birth of Jesus would symbolize recovery of a nation. Nevertheless, Jesus was handed over to the Romans on political grounds, not religious. The Jews charged Jesus with blasphemy but found him not guilty, while the Romans believed he was guilty of sedition. Although Jesus was not found guilty by the Romans he was put to death anyway, and his death launched a cultural avalanche.

Separation of Christian Church and State only started during the Protestant reformation due to Martin Luther's Doctrine of the Two Kingdoms. With separation of Church and State only rules created by man became legally binding. In a way, the situation back then resembles current tolerance of Sharia law by western cultures on their territory. Certain communities are allowed to impose their own religious laws upon their own people no matter what the legal code of the country they reside in says.

The rules imposed by the Book of Leviticus on the people of Israel can still be found in contemporary legal documents and guidelines.

It makes very good sense not to touch and eat carcasses of animals which 'died of themselves' or those not slaughtered in a controlled manner because of risk of infection and potential of spread of deadly diseases. It also seems justified to isolate those who do touch things and creatures which are 'unclean and abominable' from others, because both ignorance and willful violation of a these rules would threaten the life and health of everyone else. Does the same set of rules in literal sense apply today? Hardly. But there is no doubt about the relevance of hygiene standards including isolation of sources of potentially lethal contagious diseases and people in incubation period of deadly infectious diseases. The only difference is that food hygiene standards in food processing were transposed from a religious code, binding only for those who adhere to a particular faith, to a civil code which is legally binding for all those who reside in a respective territory.

> *Or if a soul touch any unclean thing, whether it be a carcass of an unclean beast, or a carcass of unclean cattle, or the carcass of unclean creeping things, and if it be hidden from him; he also shall be unclean, and guilty. [Leviticus, chapter 5, verse 2]*

> *Moreover the soul that shall touch any unclean thing, as the uncleanness of man, or any unclean beast, or any abominable unclean thing, and eat of the flesh of the sacrifice of peace offerings, which pertain unto the LORD, even that soul shall be cut off from his people. [Leviticus, chapter 7, verse 21]*

Our ancestors had a good reason to be scared of certain 'beasts that shall not be eaten'. It is not wise to keep pigs in areas where shortage of clean water is a continuous concern, and where contamination of this precious resource with sewage which pigs do indeed produce in very large quantity would threaten entire communities which depend on such resource. Another concern would be Trichinella spiralis, a parasite which resides in pork muscle tissue, and causes devastating disease in those who eat pork. Trichinosis would be a very good reason why people at that time did not think that pork is safe to eat. Rabbits, hares, and snakes, and creatures that 'live in water that have not fins and scales' (seafood), are now considered perfectly safe to eat providing they meet hygienic standards; and the reasons for avoiding some of them are only cultural. However, these rules did make perfect sense back then. Seafood contaminated with waste water would not be safe to eat. In addition to that there was no way how to transport and store fresh seafood safely so it would become a dangerous source of food poisonings. At more abstract level, environmental protection standards which were described in the Book of Leviticus are still relevant today. We are no longer worried about pigs spoiling our wells because we understand the risks well enough to be able to manage them; but in more abstract terms we still do worry about environmental pollution which has the potential to destroy water and soil and contaminate the food chain. The ancient code was superimposed by rules which reflect the level of knowledge people now have. Very little has changed in the sense that predators, rodents, and birds of prey are not considered edible by most cultures; and consumption of insects is limited to very few edible species which always exclude any necrophorous species. Operation rooms are divided into sterile (clean) and non-sterile (unclean) areas; and people are expected to follow hygienic standards when handling dead animals and other unclean or potentially infected materials.

These rules of cleanliness were temporarily forgotten during the Middle Ages, the Dark Age, when hygiene became a very serious problem in overpopulated urban areas. The exact content of the Bible was changing over time and inclusion and exclusion of chapters had to be approved by papal councils. The Hebrew Bible was not part of Christian religious doctrine in early Middle Ages when rejection of the Laws of Moses by Jesus was still well remembered. Should the rule on clean and unclean status of certain animal species be followed, rats and fleas would never become a problem as devastating as they were during the plague pandemic.

Apparently, medieval priests paid more attention to the part on Holy water and Hyssop and focused less on the part on washing one's body and clothes. This failure to control plague pandemic was not caused by unavailability or inaccessibility of the relevant information. It was a failure caused by group-think, persecution and elimination of ideological and scientific dissent, suppression of information sources, and general unwillingness to challenge unanimously accepted truth.

And that ye may put difference between holy and unholy, and between unclean and clean; [Leviticus, chapter 10, verse 10]

And for these ye shall be unclean: whosoever toucheth the carcass of them shall be unclean until the even. [Leviticus, chapter 11, verse 24]

And whosoever beareth ought of the carcass of them shall wash his clothes, and be unclean until the even. [Leviticus, chapter 11, verse 25]

The most dangerous contagious disease of that time was leprosy, which had to be distinguished from other illnesses with skin manifestations. Priests had the authority to isolate an 'unclean person' from others for a period of 7 days which would then be either waved or extended, depending on status of the person's health. Priests as presented in the Old Testament did have certain functions which now belong to different parts of state administration. Among other duties they had the authority to supervise population's long-term reproduction and genetic health. The phenomenon of sexual relationships within nuclear family almost certainly occurred in some communities; encouraged by relatively liberal attitude of the Romans and by the need to preserve culture and unity of a small community in hostile environment. Another motivator was important at that time just as much as it is relevant in some cultures today and that was the need to keep property within a family. The result would almost certainly be genetic degeneration caused by inbreeding which the ancient Book of Leviticus was anxious to prevent. Adultery threatened well-being and survival of a family clan. Abandoned dependents who had lost their breadwinner would have had very little chance to survive in a harsh and unforgiving world. No matter how harsh this was toward the offspring, survival of a community as a whole was unaffected by the presence of illegitimate descendants who were ostracized because of their origin and were generally utilized as slaves.

In this context, the priests not only became the guardians of morality, as they are now often perceived; their role was also to keep up long-term genetic and behavioral health of the community they looked after. They were the ones who isolated or eliminated the 'insane', the 'undisciplined', and the 'wicked'.

Nowadays, people expect doctors to treat their bodies and minds, both at individual and population level. Some cultures no longer require religious service when people enter and leave this world: at birth and at brink of death. One thing has not changed though: people still expect both doctors and priests to be the ethical pillars of society that never fall, because without them, gates of the underworld would remain unguarded.

THE RIGHTFUL AND THE WICKED

The Book of Leviticus was not completely forgotten as it may seem. Its teachings are extensively studied by some minority religious movements such as Jehovah Witnesses who base their rejection of blood transfusions on belief that blood is 'unclean'. The question of consent with treatment and the right to refuse treatment dates back to Hippocrates who had to explain the patient what the physician is going to do with his body and what measures the patient has to undertake to get healthy again. Ancient medicine is now considered paternalistic; however, it is difficult to imagine an ancient practitioner who would be enforcing any treatment on a non-compliant patient who himself or whose family had to pay the doctor directly. Major part of medicine in ancient Greece consisted of dietary adjustments, something what is impossible without patient's understanding and willing cooperation. Contagious diseases were a different matter, and patients affected by certain diseases were seriously ostracized if they did not comply with the regimen imposed upon them voluntarily. The Book of Leviticus is very specific on the rules for patients with skin diseases and those suffering from leprosy.

Patient's refusal of blood transfusion on religious grounds is one of the most controversial examples of conflict between medical ethics and religion. Jehovah Witnesses consider refusal of blood transfusions fundamental because acceptance of blood which is sacred would prevent them from entering Paradise. Members of the Church are required to observe this rule under threat of expulsion from the community. Those who accept blood and revoke this way their membership in the organization are then ostracized by the community to the point that they are completely blanked by their lifelong friends and family members who are still part of the Church, and essentially treated as outcasts. The Watchtower Society introduced the policy of refusal of blood transfusion in 1945. Since 1961 it enforced zero tolerance towards those who willfully accept blood transfusion. The number of deaths caused by refusal of blood transfusion on religious grounds is estimated around 9,000 a year. Death caused by maternal hemorrhage is about 44 times higher among Jehovah Witnesses than in general population[2]. Current medicine accepts the patient's right to refuse treatment but generally does not tolerate refusal of treatment for minors by their parents.

According to the U.S. Supreme Court decision in the case Prince vs. Massachusetts[3], parents are 'free to make martyrs of themselves; but this does not follow that they are free, in identical circumstances, to make martyrs of their children'. In practice, a hospital would ask for an order permitting administration of blood over parent's objection. Jehovah Witnesses who refuse transfusion are under significant influence of the Church, and one can argue that their decision is not fully autonomous. One-to-one talk between the patient and physician can help the patient to make an autonomous informed decision on treatment. Confidentiality between the patient and physician can make the patient more willing to accept treatment without undue influences from outside. People can and do reject cancer treatment and end-of-life medical procedures, but this is a personal choice and not a policy enforced by a Church or other authority.

Recently, Catholic Church in America attempted to enforce a ban on birth control in some states for their followers[4]. This idea sparked nation-wide debate on insurance coverage and the need of parental consent with prescription of birth control pills and consent with administration of emergency contraception and performing abortions in teenage girls. The debate on the

---

[2]   Radomyski, Mateusz. 2011. "Medical Oaths: When Religion and Ethics Collide." *Amsterdam Law Forum* 3 (1): 68–80.

[3]   *Prince vs. Massachusetts.* 1944. U.S. Supreme Court.

[4]   Chapin, Laura. 2012. "Mitt Romney and the GOP's War on Birth Control." *US News*, February 6.

implementation of rules defined in the Old Testament is ongoing and probably never ending, and there will always be more than one way of looking at the matters from individual human rights vs. population health perspectives.

THE GUIDE FOR THE PERPLEXED

Hebrew physician and philosopher Moses Maimonides, in Hebrew known as 'Rabbi Moshe Ben Maimon', or 'RaMBaM', and in Arabic literature as Abu 'Imran Musa ben Maimun ibn 'Abd Allah. Maimonides was born in the Spanish city of Cordoba in 1135 and died in Fostat (Cairo) in Egypt in 1204. Moses was only thirteen years old when Cordoba fell into the hands of fanatical Almohades, and his family was forced into exile where they led a nomadic life for twelve years. In 1160 they settled at Fez, pretending to be Moslems. Maimonides' reputation of a physician was steadily growing and this made him more visible to the authorities which even charged him with the crime of having relapsed from Islam. In 1165 Maimonides' family left for Acre, continued to Jerusalem, and then to Fostat (Cairo), where they settled. He made a living as a physician and authored ten medical works including the Oath of Maimonides. He gained fame mainly from his work on Jewish law, chiefly the 'Book of the Commandments'[5], 'The Pentateuch'; 'Commentary on the Mishnah'[6]; 'The Law in Review'[7]; and masterpiece written in Arabic 'The Guide to the Perplexed'[8] in which he tried to address apparent disparity between biblical and scientific and philosophical ideas for the readers of the Torah. This effort to apply rational thinking was not always met with understanding. Denounced to Church authorities by Jewish adversaries, the first and most thematic volume of Maimonides'

---

[5]   Maimonides, Moses. 1204. *The Book of the Commandments: Kitab Al-Fara'id (Sefer Ha-Mitzvot).*

[6]   Maimonides, Moses. 1204. *Commentary of the Mishnah: Kitab Al-Siraj (Sefer Ha-Maor, Perush Ha-Mishnah).*

[7]   Maimonides, Moses. 1204. *Mishneh Torah (The Law in Review).*

[8]   Maimonides, Moses. 1204. *The Guide for the Perplexed.* Translated from the original Arabic text by M. Friedlander in 1904.

code, the *Sefer ha-Mada (Book of Knowledge)*, was burnt at Montpellier in 1232, along with The Guide to the Perplexed[9]. In the Guide for the Perplexed, Maimonides pays lot of attention not only to philosophical issues of that time with regards to deity; but also explains rationale behind the Book of Leviticus and its practical implications on daily life and on medical practice:

> *Males or females that are unclean through running issue, and a woman after childbirth, must in addition bring a sacrifice, because their uncleanness occurs less frequently than that of women in their separation. All these cases of uncleanliness, viz., running issue of males or females, menstruations, leprosy, dead bodies of human beings, carcasses of beasts and creeping things, and issue of semen, are sources of dirt and filth. We have thus shown that the above precepts are very useful in many respects. First, they keep us at a distance from dirty and filthy objects: secondly, they guard the Sanctuary; thirdly, they pay regard to an established custom (for the Sabeans submitted to very troublesome restrictions when unclean, as you will soon hear): fourthly, they lightened that burden for us; for we are not impeded through these laws in our ordinary occupations by the distinction the Law makes between that which is unclean and that which is clean. (The Guide for the Perplexed, p 524)*

> *Another custom among the Sabeans, which is still widespread, is this: whatever is separated from the body, as hair, nail, or blood, is unclean; every barber is therefore unclean in their estimation, because he touches blood and hair; whenever a person passes a razor over his skin he must take a bath in running water." (The Guide for the Perplexed, p 525)*

Compliance with this practice would have made a fundamental difference during the plague epidemic because it would mean isolation of people who 'come in contact with unclean animals such as rats', and, more importantly, would introduce hygienic practices for those who get in contact with 'whatever is separated from the body' should it be blood, issue, or any other surgically removed or opened structure. This rule effectively described principles of clean surgery.

---

[9]   Islamic Philosophy Online, Inc. n.d. "The Muslim Philosophy."

Blood (Lev. xvii. 12), and nebelah, i.e., the flesh of an animal that died of itself (Deut. xiv. 21), are indigestible, and injurious as food: Trejah, an animal in a diseased state (Exod. xxii. 30), is on the way of becoming a nebelah. (The Guide for the Perplexed, p 528)

The commandment concerning the killing of animals is necessary, because the natural food of man consists of vegetables and of the flesh of animals: the best meat is that of animals permitted to be used as food. No doctor has any doubts about this. Since, therefore, the desire of procuring good food necessitates the slaying of animals, the Law enjoins that the death of the animal should be the easiest. It is not allowed to torment the animal by cutting the throat in a clumsy manner, by pole axing, or by cutting off a limb whilst the animal is alive. It is also prohibited to kill an animal with its young on the same day (Lev. xxii. 28), in order that people should be restrained and prevented from killing the two together in such a manner that the young is slain in the sight of the mother; for the pain of the animals under such circumstances is very great. There is no difference in this case between the pain of man and the pain of other living beings, since the love and tenderness of the mother for her young ones is not produced by reasoning, but by imagination, and this faculty exists not only in man but in most living beings. This law applies only to ox and lamb, because of the domestic animals used as food these alone are permitted to us, and in these cases the mother recognizes her young. (The Guide for the Perplexed, p 528-9)

E.g., bodily exercise, in its different kinds, is necessary for the proper preservation of health in the opinion of him who understands the science of medicine; writing is considered as very useful by scholars. (The Guide for the Perplexed, p 448)

The comment above reminds people of the duty to treat humanely animals which are slain for food. The Book of Leviticus as explained and presented by Maimonides did not require obedience without a reason. All measures described in the Hebrew Bible in his eyes had rational justification. There are many practices which are described in the text below which were forgotten in the coming centuries because they were considered heretical. As per Maimonides, good diet and exercise are the most important conditions of good health; and medicine to be effective shall be based on observation and experiment. Maimonides clearly rejected astrology which he compared to witchcraft, having no sympathy for this pseudoscience. This is the book which was burned by the Christians at Montpelier in 1232, along with many other 'heretical texts'.

> *[The Law prohibits] everything that the idolaters, according to their doctrine, and contrary to reason, consider as being useful and acting in the manner of certain mysterious forces. Comp. 'Neither shall ye walk in their ordinances' (Lev. xviii. 3) and 'Ye shall not walk in the manners of the nation which I cast out before you' (ibid. xx. 23). Our Sages call such acts 'the ways of the Amorite': they are kinds of witchcraft, because they are not arrived at by reason, but are similar to the performances of witchcraft, which is necessarily connected with the influences of the stars; thus ['the manners of the nations'] lead people to extol, worship, and praise the stare. Our Sages say distinctly, 'whatever is used as medicine' does not come under the law of 'the ways of the Amorite': tor they hold that only such cures as are recommended by reason are permitted, and other cures are prohibited. (The Guide for the Perplexed, p 481-2)*

> *The uterus of animals which have been selected for the Sanctuary must be buried; it must not be suspended from a tree, and not buried in the cross-road, because this is one of 'the ways of the Amorite.' Hence you may learn how to treat similar cases. It is not inconsistent that a nail of the gallows and the tooth of a fox have been permitted to be used as cures: for these things have been considered in those days as facts established by experiment. They served as cures, in the same manner as the hanging of the peony over a person subject to epileptic fits, or the application of a dog's refuse to the swellings of the throat, and of the vapors of vinegar and marcasite to the swelling of hard tumors. **For the Law permits as medicine everything that has been verified by experiment, although it cannot be explained by analogy.** (The Guide for the Perplexed, p 482)*

> *Of the letters written after the completion of the 'Guide,' the one addressed to the wise men of Marseilles (1194) is especially*

noteworthy. Maimonides was asked to give his opinion on astrology. He regretted in his reply that they were not yet in the possession of his Mishneh Torah; they would have found in it the answer to their question. According to his opinion, man should only believe what he can grasp with his intellectual faculties, or perceive by his senses, or what he can accept on trustworthy authority. Beyond this nothing should be believed. **Astrological statements, not being founded on any of these three sources of knowledge, must be rejected.** *He had himself studied astrology, and was convinced that it was no science at all. (The Guide for the Perplexed, p 21)*

In Egypt, the family no longer had to hide their Jewish faith, and Maimonides gained fame as a physician. Famous Muslim military leader Sultan Saladin and his son al-Afdal were among his patients among many other high profile figures of that time. His influence on Judaism extended to the larger world; and his philosophical texts influenced great medieval Scholastic writers, and even later thinkers, such as Benedict de Spinoza and G.W. Leibniz. His medical writings constitute a significant chapter in the history of medical science. According to 20th century historian Waldemar Schweisheimer[10], Maimonides' medical teachings are not antiquated at all; in fact they are astonishingly modern in tone and contents.

---

[10]   Bokser, Rabbi Ben Zion. 2013. "Moses Maimonides." *Encyclopedia Britannica.*

II. THE BLACK DEATH

The two plague pandemics which ravaged Europe in 6th and 14th centuries inflicted enormous numbers of casualties and caused profound changes in society ranging from philosophical to economic. Corpses infected with plague were used during the Mongol attack on Caffa in 1346. Although this incident effectively started the 14th century plague pandemic it was not its cause. Plague is still considered a potential weapon which could be utilized by terrorists; and contingencies are planned for the eventuality of an attack or spontaneous outbreak. Conditions which were necessary for escalation of local outbreak to a pandemic were numerous, and included overpopulation, lack of hygienic standards, elimination of ideological and scientific dissent, suppression of information which did not conform to the only authorized life-science doctrine, elimination of any alternative ideas and life-science doctrines together with their proponents, exclusion of the Hebrew Bible from religious teachings, and most importantly loss of autonomy of the subjugated populations as the core causes. Group-think was the result of several centuries lasting systematic elimination of critical thinkers who were the only people who had the capacity to recognize true nature of the disease, and find a way of stopping the pandemic.

Plague, a disease known already to the Pharaohs, swept through Europe in 14th century and claimed 25 million lives in the first wave and another 25 million in those which followed. The same disease, now recognized as the Justinian Plague, ravaged Byzantine Empire in 541-542 AD and claimed about 25 million lives in the Middle East and Eastern Mediterranean. This was very considerable part of the population and the worst pandemic on record. *Yersinia pestis*[11], Gram-negative bacteria with typical safety pin appearance, is primarily a rodent pathogen. Humans get infected when bitten by a rat flea which carries the bacteria in its guts where the microbes multiply. When feeding on animal or human blood, fleas

---

[11]   Bednar, Marek, Vera Frankova, Jiri Schindler, Andrej Soucek, and Jiri Vavra. 1996. *Lekarska Mikrobiologie*. Marvil.

regurgitate part of the blood they have in their stomachs including the pathogen, and transfer the infection to the host. While growing in the flea, *Yersinia pestis* loses its capsular layer which is its main protection against phagocytosis by macrophages. When transferred to animals or humans, most of the bacteria are killed by the immune system, but some are taken up by tissue macrophages which are unable to kill them and provide protected environment for the organisms to synthesize their virulence factors. A macrophage then serves like a Trojan horse for the pathogen. Upon release, *Yersinia pestis* quickly spreads to regional lymph nodes which become swollen, tender, and hot. These massively enlarged lymph nodes are responsible for main symptom of bubonic form of plague, the characteristic buboes. Within hours of the initial flea bite, the pathogen spreads in the bloodstream and affects liver, spleen, and lung tissue.

Whilst untreated bubonic form of plague has mortality about 50 to 60% of patients, pulmonary form and plague septicemia are nearly 100% fatal. Apart from the typical buboes, the symptoms include high fever and chills, general malaise, headaches and body aches, and vomiting and nausea. Pulmonary form causes people to cough bloody sputum in severe fits. Plague septicemia is so fast that people do not develop the typical buboes before they die. Plague gets transferred from infected rats to humans through fleas which serve as a vector of the disease, and then, as the epidemic progresses to its pulmonary form spreads from one person to another[12].

---

[12]   Chamberlain, Neal R. 2010. "Lymphoreticular and Hematopoetic Infections: Plague."

THE JUSTINIAN PLAGUE

The oldest epidemic of plague was recorded in ancient Egypt[13]. Archeologist Panagiotakopulu searched burial sites for remains of insects and small rodents to find out what diseases ancient populations might have had, and discovered a plague infested flea. Black rat was endemic to India and spread to ancient Egypt on board of merchant ships. For plague to move from rodents to humans and cause an epidemic or pandemic, the sylvatic brown and gray rats which otherwise stay in the wild need to come into contact with black rat or people themselves. Panagiotakopulu believes that the main impulse which forced Nile rats and their plague-infested fleas to move closer to human settlements and share environment with people were periodic floods. Contact between sylvatic and urban rat populations was possible due to existence of grain silos and storage sites in which both rat types exchanged fleas and ultimately spread plague to humans. Ebers Papyrus, medical text written about 1500 B.C., describes an epidemic of a disease which looks like bubonic plague. Although in the ancient world plague was a well-known disease, it mostly caused localized outbreaks which were self-limiting - until the pandemic of 541.

Justinian Plague is believed to have been imported either from Ethiopia or Egypt, where plague was present in sylvatic form among population of brown, gray, and black rats. The disease likely spread to Europe on the backs of shipboard black rats which carried plague-infested fleas. Subsequent epidemics which followed in 6th, 7th, and 8th century, were more localized and less deadly, but caused so much disruption that eventually led to demise of the Byzantine Empire. Based on the accounts of Procopius, a 6th century historian, the origin of Justinian plague can be traced to the port of Pelusium where it was first reported in 541 AD. From Pelusium it spread to Alexandria and throughout Egypt, and consequently in 542 through Constantinople to Asia Minor, Greece, Italy, France, Spain, and

---

[13]   Walker, Cameron. 2004. "Bubonic Plague Traced to Ancient Egypt." *National Geographic News.*

eventually north into the British Isles. Orent[14] in her book on the history future of plague argues that although Justinian I was not responsible for creating the disease, he created conditions which allowed the pandemic to break out. Until then, plague did exist in urban settings but its outbreaks were localized. The pandemic followed the movements of men and goods in Justinian's resurrected Roman Empire and was essentially the consequence of imperial overstretch, and globalization of economy and centralization of vital resources.[15]

> *Without the empire, the bread dole, the huge shipments of grain and clothes from Africa, it is difficult to imagine how the First Pandemic could ever have erupted. (Orent, 2004)*

As per Procopius, the 6th century citizens of Constantinople suffered from shortage of food as a result of an extended period of cold weather and low sunshine, and were therefore weakened and prone to disease. This mini nuclear winter is believed to have been caused either by a comet hitting the earth or the eruption of a massive volcano[16]. This climatic anomaly affected the harvests and ability of the locals to achieve self-sufficiency in basic food supply; and many of the inhabitants, especially the poor, were becoming dependent on bread dole. Marjolein Schat in her paper 'Justinian's Foreign Policy and the Plague: Did Justinian Create the First Pandemic?' explains how huge warehouses and bread dole in Justinian's Empire created the plague pandemics of 541:

> *The grain tribute from Africa was approximately 240 metric tons per year (Evans 1996) and primarily went to Constantinople where it was used in a bread dole to feed the people of the city. The grain was brought to Constantinople by ship across the*

---

[14]   Orent, Wendy. 2012. *Plague: The Mysterious Past and Terrifying Future of the World's Most Dangerous Disease*. Free Pres.

[15]   Walker, Cameron. 2004. "Bubonic Plague Traced to Ancient Egypt." *National Geographic News*.

[16]   Walker, Cameron. 2004. "Bubonic Plague Traced to Ancient Egypt." *National Geographic News*.

Mediterranean Sea. Bad weather and heavy seas closed the Mediterranean Sea to shipping from November to March, and it was still dangerous an additional two months on either side of the closed period (Temin 2001). With only four "safe" months out of a year in which grain could be shipped, horrea (warehouses) were built to store the grain. The early horrea of Ostia and Rome were 60 foot by 100 foot one storey buildings (Vitelli 1980), but in Constantinople some have been reported as large as 90 feet by 280 feet and "ineffably" tall (Evans 1996). The horrea were ideal breeding grounds for rats and fleas, and Orent (2004) claims that the combination of these plague factories and expanded trade routes were the catalyst for the plague going from an outbreak to epidemic and then to pandemic. (Ibid)

Important factor which contributed to spread of the Justinian Plague was gradual but profound loss of individual freedoms which came with feudalism. Consequent loss of autonomy resulted in loss of ability to employ protective measures at individual level. Increasing dependence of the most vulnerable part of the population on bread dole facilitated the spread of plague from infected horrea to people who had no other options but to take what was given to them. Another important factor was the spread of Christianity which was in its early stages based on series of dogmas which could not be challenged. Causal factors of the medieval plague, the so-called 'unholy trinity' were bacterium Yersinia pestis as a pathogen, the black rat as a reservoir, and a flea as a vector. Without these three factors present all at once no outbreak can occur. But not even these factors together would cause a pandemic by themselves because they require other conditions to manifest full force. The essential conditions are existence of a reservoir of sylvatic population of infected rodents; existence of population of urban or shipyard rodents; place where the two populations come in close contact to allow transfer of infected fleas between the two populations which are normally separate; contact between people and fleas from infected rodents or via infected fleas once the rodents had been disposed of; and eventually during later phases of the epidemic through direct contact between infected people and contact with dead corpses and their belongings and clothes. During the Justinian Plague, infected rats were imported on board ships and their introduction into naive environment and contact with sylvatic rats created a reservoir which would cause subsequent series of outbreaks in the following decades. Contact between infected rats and fleas in grain silos was one route of transmission, the other being transfer from infected fleas hiding in clothes to people who were handling the shipments. So far the pathogenesis is clear as presented in mainstream literature but the story does not seem to be complete just yet because 19th and 20th century bubonic plague outbreaks have completely different dynamics than the medieval form. The medieval Black Death pandemic was not an inevitable disaster caused by adversity of nature but a combination of natural factors and man-made conditions which allowed it to become as deadly as it was. Essential condition for a plague outbreak is a contact with reservoir. If the local population of sylvatic rats is already infected, the essential condition required is the contact between sylvatic and urban population of rats which then come in contact with domestic animals and people. Expanded shipping routes which reach reservoirs further away increase the probability that a reservoir will eventually be reached. Under any other circumstances, if there were any alternative trade routes outside plague infested regions, the fact of reaching a reservoir would be a mere aggravating condition of the pandemic. But because there were no alternatives, and the empire could not cope without supply of essential commodities from North Africa, the relationship between plague-infested regions and the Byzantine Empire became that of a cause and effect because of strategic dependence of the Empire on clothes and grains from North Africa. Single point of entry (Constantinople) then played the role of a critical condition because the port could not be shut down. From Constantinople the infection got into the local supply through horrea and due to the bread dole it was pushed to people who had no way of avoiding the infected material. Due to outbound shipping it was spread globally to other ports. At the same time, the population was becoming impoverished and unable to employ even the most basic precautions to protect themselves against spread of the disease. Long wars abroad sucked up resources which were desperately needed elsewhere. This lack of capacity to cope at individual level was worsened by lack of investment in public infrastructure such as baths and waste management, and lack of capacity or will to improve the living standard of the population.

Causes and conditions of the plague pandemic

Causal factors	Plague	
Presence of a causative agent: bacterium **Yersinia pestis**	} 'Unholy trinity'	
Presence of a primary host: **rats**		
Presence of a vector: **fleas**		
Conditions	**Outbreak** → **Epidemic**	→ **Pandemic**
Existence of a **reservoir**: sylvatic population of infected rodents	Y (essential)[17]	All essential factors have to be present to produce an outbreak. ↓ Multiple unprotected routes ☐ multiple ways o transfer ☐ tautology[18]
Existence of a population of **urban or shipyard rats**	Y (essential)	
Presence of an **infected vector (flea)**	Y (essential)	

[17]   Y (essential) = necessary conditions which have to be present all at the same time to produce an outbreak, not sufficient by itself. If any of these conditions is missing, the outbreak does not occur.

[18]   Tautology: if any of 1-n variables is true, X will happen. Probability of X happening increases with number of variables.

Causal factors	**Plague**	
Conditions	**Outbreak** → **Epidemic**	→ **Pandemic**
Contact between susceptible human and infected rats (A)	Y (optional – either of A conditions)	All essential factors have to be present to produce an outbreak.
Contact between susceptible human and infected flea (A)	Y (optional – either of A conditions)	↓
Contact between susceptible and infected human ^causative agent capable of transfer via direct contact (A)	Y (optional – either of A conditions)	Multiple unprotected routes ways of transfer ☐ tautology[19]
Handling dead bodies[20] (presence of an infected vector is required, e.g. fleas on clothes ☐ animals feeding on infected flesh)	Y (strengthens effect of other A conditions) **OUTBREAK** ☐**EPIDEMIC** ☐**PANDEMIC**	

Causative agent + vectors + susceptible host + (any of A) conditions => outbreak

Causative agent + vectors + susceptible host + (all of A) conditions => epidemic or pandemic

---

[19]   Tautology: if any of 1-n variables is true, X will happen. Probability of X happening increases with number of variables.

[20]   Broughton, Methew J. 2014. "Catapulted Death: Can a Flying Corpse Distribute the Plague?" *Insects, Disease, and History.*

In ancient times, the infection killed nearly 100% of all infected patients and spread at enormous speed, roughly the same distance a day as current plague in a year. During the World War Two Japanese physician Ishii Shiro from Unit 731 in Japanese occupied Manchuria experimented with bubonic plague for its potential to be used as bacteriological warfare. When the war was over, thousands of plague and tularemia-infected rats were released in the wild. The disease did not spread like medieval plague but was largely self-limiting. It is likely that the bacterium mutated as well and over the centuries lost its main virulence factors.

Susceptibility to the disease is another factor to be considered because the survivors acquire lifelong immunity which protects them from subsequent outbreaks. In addition, certain genotypes are more resilient to the disease than others. This natural resistance was caused by a mutation which some researchers believe is the same as mutation CCR-5 Delta 32 which prevents the pathogen from entering macrophages and is responsible for resistance against HIV. This allele is unique to European population and is not at all present in Asia, India and the Middle East; places which were ravaged by medieval plague the same way or even more than Europe. Whether there is a connection between mutations in this particular gene and the selection pressure caused by the medieval plague pandemic remains unanswered[21].

---

[21]   Cohn, SK, and LT Weaver. 2006. "The Black Death and AIDS: CCR5-32 in Genetics and History." *QJM* 99 (8): 497–503.

Causes and conditions which led to the Justinian plague

Expanded shipping routes reaching other reservoirs	Y - **Essential condition** in absence of causal factors AND aggravating condition if causal factors are already present	Y - essential condition for creation of pandemic: absence of alternatives AND presence of conditions for epidemic
Economy of an empire dependent on trade with remote places, supply of essential commodities (grain and clothes) from North Africa to a single port creating **strategic dependence**	Y – **Cause and effect**. Dependence on causal factor AND aggravating condition	
Imperial overreach → high taxes imposed to cover war expenses and ambitious building projects which sucked up resources and impoverished local population → **loss of autonomy** (B)	Y (optional – either of B conditions)	Y – inability to take precautions at individual level
Lack of investment in public infrastructure (baths) →lowering standard of hygiene including pest control (B)	Y (optional – either of B conditions)	Y – weakening of defenses at multiple levels
Bread dole → dependence on the ruler: inability of local population to find alternative sources / move due to reported poverty → **changes towards feudalism** → entrapment of population at risk: loss of autonomy AND existential dependence	Y (optional – either of B conditions)	Y – inability to take precautions at individual level (true for most of Europe)

THE 1348 PLAGUE

But the worst was still to come. European culture forgot about its roots and entered a period which is now called the Dark Ages. Religious fundamentalism engulfed Europe and kept its inhabitants in submission, obedient and compliant. Medical science degenerated from Hippocratic concept of empirical learning and respect to nature and life to a very abstract way of explaining the origin of human illness and suffering as consequence of the wrath of God. Astrology, a science which was once by Maimonides described as backwards pseudoscience was now becoming mainstream life-science.

The authority to provide treatment to individuals and population as a whole shifted from physicians to priests once again. Many books were burned; many lessons learned in the past the hard way were forgotten and replaced with religious doctrines. In 1346, pestilence once again spread throughout Europe; this time from Crimea, where it probably broke out as the result of biological warfare attack during the Siege of Caffa[22]. Mark Wheeling in his paper refers to Gabriele Mussi's memoir in which the onset of deadly disease is described in great detail. Tartars and Saracens who were coming in large numbers from the East were falling ill with a deadly disease which was unknown in the area at that time and resembled bubonic plague. The Mongol army hurled large numbers of plague-infected cadavers into the besieged Crimean city of Caffa, disposing off of corpses and transmitting the disease to the inhabitants. Consequently, the fleeing survivors of the siege spread plague from Caffa to the Mediterranean Basin. Mussi also mentioned that the Italians fleeing from Caffa spread the disease to other Italian ports. Crimea is widely accepted as the origin of the 13th century plague outbreak in Europe. Even though the Siege of Caffa was one of the points of entry, according to Wheeling it was not a decisive one. There were many other routes which allowed spreading of the Black Death, mainly through merchant ships which always had enough

---

[22]   Wheelis, Mark. 2002. "Biological Warfare at the 1346 Siege of Caffa." *Emerg Infect Dis [serial Online]*, September 2002.

rats on board. Killing off the rats on board ships made the situation even worse, because hungry fleas started feeding on human blood and spread the disease even faster. With incubation period 2 to 6 days, infection during unloading of goods full of fleas would allow enough time to spread the plague to yet another port.

From Crimea, plague spread to Constantinople, Asia Minor, Cyprus, Crete, Sicily, Sardinia, Corsica, and Marseille which it reached in January 1348. By June the same year, it continued spreading through North African ports, swept through Greece, the Balkans, Venice and Papal States, Castile, and Aragon to France and all the way to Normandy, and then through Calais to Bristol and London. Alps and the Pyrenees did not stop the plague. Interestingly, Danube lowlands which had extensive trade with Crimea, too, were only affected by plague which was spreading from the South in late 1949 and 1950, and not directly from Crimea. By 1349, plague pandemic affected most of England and Wales, Southern part of Scotland and Ireland, Western Castile and Portugal, Southern part of Norway, Rhine and Danube lowlands, and eventually in 1350 remaining part of northern and eastern Europe around the Baltic and all the way to Russian steppe. Only Poland was spared and apparently suffered very few deaths[23].

Causes of the 1348 plague pandemic

The plague pandemic is the worst natural disaster on record. It has been extensively studied by scholars not only for its dynamics and social changes it triggered, but also for the unique psychological effects. Medicine of those days was unable to pinpoint the cause of the disease, and with the philosophy it was using to understand the pandemic it could have never come to the right conclusion and effective defense. Philosophical concept of medieval medicine is so different from current understanding of natural sciences and human body, that its disconnection from reality is difficult to comprehend. Medieval institutions faced the horrors of Black Death with apathy and fatalism, only providing palliative therapy to themselves and the subjects they were supposed to care for; like if there was nothing what could have been done to stop the plague.

---

[23]   Luebke, David M. n.d. "The Spread of Plague."

Looking back at the measures described in the Book of Leviticus, the oldest book on epidemiology and hygiene on record, one has to wonder how is it possible that these teachings were not used to combat the disease. Rats and fleas were unclean under this code and people were not supposed to come in any contact with them. Medieval teachings considered bathing great threat to human health, in the difference from the Romans for whom bathing was not only part of personal hygiene but also an opportunity to socialize. The Book of Leviticus required the unclean to wash their bodies and clothes, and burn items which could not be cleaned, in order to have a living quarters pronounced clean again. Was this experience completely forgotten? This seems unlikely, because the Bible was extensively studied by then scholars. Somehow, the message from the Hebrew Bible either was not passed down or was not understood during the 13th century plague epidemic. It may be difficult to claim with confidence that the rules for isolation of patients with leprosy and measures against rats and fleas would have helped to control the pandemic, or at least slow down its speed. However, the major conditions which were crucial to uncontrollable spread of this pandemic are easy to identify.

Medieval scholarship after the First renaissance did refer back to the teachings of ancient philosophers but the understanding of these texts was not the same as that of ancient Greeks. Hippocrates's texts are characteristic by attitude which emphasizes nature over philosophy and observation over theoretical dogmas and abstract reasoning. The same applies to Maimonides whose reasoning was very rational. Medieval medicine diverted from these principles substantially and put philosophy and complex theoretical structures first, even when they were in direct contradiction with observations. Discrepancies were then explained through sophisticated theories whilst the dogmatic theoretical foundation was never questioned. As a result of divorce of science from empirical experience and observation, medieval medicine lacked capacity to understand biological nature of disease. Christian anti-Semitism resulted in substantial change in understanding of the Hebrew Bible, including the Book of Leviticus. If any parts of the Hebrew Bible were used the focus was on purely theoretical and dogmatic scholarship rather than practical advice from the Code.

During the Middle Ages, it was illegal for all but the Church to own, study and interpret the Scriptures. Moreover, not all Scriptures which are included in the Bible today were part of it back then. Disagreements over canonicity of books such as Hebrew, James, Peter, and Revelation were settled through Church councils and papal pronouncements.[24] Many Jewish physicians became victims of anti-Semitic pogroms. One of the most prominent Jewish doctors who were forced to flee the country in which he lived and practiced was Moses Maimonides, the author of ten medical works which included the Oath of Maimonides and the Guide for the Perplexed[25].

It is not a coincidence that the plague which ravaged Europe in 13th century followed after expulsion of the only medical practitioners who had knowledge of the Hebrew Bible which provided at least some rational guidance. Elimination of free thinkers as bearers of competing ideologies as a 'threat to the establishment' thus has causal relationship to the later limitations of the society with regards to understanding of causes and pathogenesis of plague. Moses Maimonides in his Guide for the Perplexed, which was written around 1190 and circulated in Arabic and Hebrew at time when he and his family already had fled Spain and settled in Egypt, argued that 'Astrology is no science at all' and therefore cannot be used as an explanation of origins of a disease. Even though the work was not accepted as given truth by the whole Jewish community, its impact was still very significant; and it was only burnt by the Christian establishment together with some other 'heretical' texts in 1232, three decades after his death. Official explanation of medieval establishment on cause of the plague pandemic was that it was the result of 'conjunction of planets'. Stove-piping, group-think and victimization, persecution, and elimination of academic, scientific, and religious dissent created an environment in which people were unwilling and unable to voice alternative opinions within the Church and Academia even if the source materials were available. The result was development of a

---

[24]   Youell, Greg. 2003. "The Bible and the Catholic Church." *Bible Research*.

[25]   "Torah Class: Rediscovering the Old Testament. Lesson 1, Introduction to Leviticus Part 1." 2014. *Old Testament Studies*. Accessed May 4.

single, dominant, supposedly perfect and ultimately unchallengeable theory of life. Few people wish to be burned alive for heresy if the other option is to pursue a good career. Feudal regimes of medieval Europe created a world in which the inhabitants lacked all means of defense against the Black Death.

The 1348 plague pandemic

Feudalist economy no longer recognized some individual rights (partially reinstituted by Magna Carta, at least in England) → **loss of autonomy** (B)	Y (optional – either of B conditions)	Y – inability & unwillingness to impose protective measures at governance level ^ inability to take precautions at individual level
Eleven years into the Hundred years war (expenses) → lack of investment in public infrastructure (hygiene and pest control) (B) → increased taxes ^ drop in living standard (B)	Y (optional – either of B conditions)	
Attack in Caffa (intentional spread of infection through large number of infected corpses thrown into a seized city)[26]	Y – a freak event	N – attack of this kind occurred only in Caffa

[26] Wheelis, Mark. 2002. "Biological Warfare at the 1346 Siege of Caffa." *Emerg Infect Dis [serial Online]*

THE ROLE OF IDEOLOGY

Loss of autonomy of subjects in feudal European states contributed to the pandemic through total loss of control over quality of services provided by medical practitioners. Any influence over this profession was only exercised through the ruler and through the Church and was not necessarily consistent with the interests of subjects in their care. Second Renaissance reintroduced ideas of ancient Greece in their original form. The concept of free will and human rights was unknown in early medieval Europe, including British Isles.

FLAWED LIFE SCIENCE DOCTRINE AS THE CAUSE OF INABILITY TO CONTAIN PLAGUE

Access to information limited to those with privileged access and ability to read (ban on possession of the Bible by all but Church, no access to scientific texts) (X)	Y – cause and effect (X)[27]	Y – No capacity to comprehend nature of the disease by **elimination of bearers of ideas, texts, and thinking people.**
Ignoring existing knowledge for ideological and dogmatic reasons (anti-Semitism, exclusion of Hebrew Bible) (X)	Y – cause and effect (X)	Essential knowledge did already exist on the subject but was not used due to internal constraints.
Exclusion of vast segments of population from education based on social status → further limitation of access based on willingness to comply with official doctrine → extreme measures taken against heretics (X)	Y – cause and effect (X)	

---

[27] Cause and effect: causal relationship between measures taken by the establishment against a "threat" (ideas, texts, and thinking people or people with certain skills) and their absence in the environment. Employment of measures X(1-n) causes absence of (means) essential for correct identification of causal relationships (links between the disease and its causes) and consequently successful management of the crisis.

Several waves of **expulsion** of Jewish scholars and physicians → **elimination of competing ideologies** (X)	Y – cause and effect (X)
→ **inability to correctly identify cause of the disease**	Y – critical condition for creation of pandemic →
Spreading of disinformation as the only "official interpretation" of religious and philosophical texts	Y – cause and effect (X)
Enforcing a single "life science" doctrine across the whole Christian world	Y – cause and effect (X)
→ **Persecution and victimization of "heretics"**, "false prophets" and free thinkers for acquiring information from unapproved sources, cogitating on it, and writing their thoughts	Y – cause and effect (X)
→ **Delusion** of whole generations of philosophers and physicians with regards to (non)existing links between cause and effect vs. mere association or no association[28]	Y – cause and effect (X)

All people were subject to the will of Almighty God, the king, and the clergy. At least in England, this was about to change with the signature of Magna Carta in 1215 and the creation of British Parliament in 1237. The Charter was confirmed many more times during the 13th century; the most significant occasion was in 1297, when the text was entered on the statute roll, giving it the status

---

[28] Moses Maimonides: The Guide for the Perplexed, 1190. "Astrology is no science at all" vs. official explanation from 1348 "Plague is caused by conjunction of planets"

of a parliamentary statute. In 1302, a group of 80 landless farm laborers at Barton upon Humber in north Lincolnshire attempted to impose a local minimum wage and stop certain restrictive practices[29]. The impact of this Charter probably would have been much less if it was not for peasant rebellions caused by the Black Death. The concept of free will and human rights was unknown in early medieval Europe, including British Isles. All people were subject to the will of Almighty God, the king, and the clergy. At least in England, this was about to change with the signature of Magna Carta in 1215 and the creation of British Parliament in 1237. The Charter was confirmed many more times during the 13th century; the most significant occasion was in 1297, when the text was entered on the statute roll, giving it the status of a parliamentary statute. The impact of this Charter probably would have been much less if it was not for peasant rebellions caused by the Black Death.

At the beginning of the Hundred Years War in 1337, actual campaigning started when the King invaded France in 1339 and laid claim to the throne of France. Following a sea victory at Sluys in 1340, Edward overran Brittany in 1342 and in 1346 he landed in Normandy, defeating the French King, Philip VI, at the Battle of Crécy. At time of the plague outbreak in England, in 1948, Edward III founded the Order of the Garter[30]. Eleven years into the Hundred Years War, in January 1348, the Black Death entered England. The first wave of Black Death hit Southern England in 1348 and during the following year it swept through Midlands and Wales to southern parts of Scotland and across the Irish Sea to Ireland.[31] The average death rate was between 30 – 45%.

In winter 1348 plague mutated in its more malignant pneumonic form, and by 1360 it became gender and age specific. Whilst the first pestilence of 1348-50 mostly affected adults, the second wave which ravaged the British Isles in early 1360's mostly killed young boys. Another wave which came in 1370's caused especially high

[29]   The National Archives. 2014. "Medieval Concept of Human Rights 1215-1500." *The National Archives.*

[30]   "Edward III (1327-1377)." 2014. *The Official Website of the British Monarchy.*

[31]   Ibeji, Mike. 2011. "Black Death." *BBC History.*

death rates among children. By 1370's, the population of England was halved, and did not start recovering until mid-1500's. Black Death pandemic which caused 50 million deaths in 14th century Europe resulted in profound social, economic, and cultural change. Contributing factors to severity of this pandemic were overpopulation, poor standard of hygiene, close contact between humans and animals, and shortage of food caused by extended period of cold weather, now known as the little ice age. The immediate economic impact of high death toll caused by plague was profound. Much of land remained deserted; landlords had difficulties finding tenants and laborers for their holdings. Wages significantly increased due to shortage of workforce, and many innovative techniques emerged to compensate for shortage of people who had to improvise.

Art completely changed form and reflected ubiquitous presence of death. In response to high death rate among bishops and priests, the Bishop of Bath and Wells released an appeal that stated:

> *On the verge of death, if they cannot have a duly ordained priest, they shall in some way make confession to each other...even to a layman, or, in default of him, to a woman.*

A good death meant reunion with Christ, while a bad death meant eternal suffering in the fires of hell. The numbers of dead became so vast that the pope resorted to consecrating the Rhone River; in which the bodies were interred[32]. Probably the most widely accepted theory about the origin of plague of the time was the one released on October 6, 1348, by the medical faculty at the University of Paris, one of the most respected institutions of that time. The statement was released upon the request of Philip VI, king of France. The report explained the plague as a result of conjunction of planets and cited authorities such as Hippocrates, Ptolemy, Albertus Magnus, and Artistotle:

> *The distant and first cause of this pestilence was and is a certain configuration in the heavens. In the year of our Lord 1345...there was a major conjunction of three higher planets in Aquarius.*

---

[32]   Des Ormeaux, AL. 2007. "The Black Death and Its Effect on Fourteen and Fifteen Century Art." Graduate Faculty of the Louisiana State University and Agricultural and Mechanical College.

Indeed, this conjunction...being the present cause of the ruinous corruption of the air that is all around us, is a harbinger of mortality and famine.

We believe that the present epidemic or plague originated from air that was corrupt in its substance...air, which is pure and clear by nature, does not putrefy or become corrupt unless it is mixed up with something else, that is, with evil vapors...[which] have come about through the configurations [of the planets], the aforesaid universal and distant cause. (Ibid)

This is exactly the type of explanation which was once condemned by Maimonides in his Guide for the Perplexed, a medical and philosophical text which was among those burned a century ago. At the time of Black Death epidemic, very little was known about the disease itself and there was no cure. The teachings of Ancient Greece could not be used in their original form because of fear of being expelled from Church for heresy. Hippocratic medicine, based on keen observation and detailed knowledge of human anatomy and physiology, would likely be able to cope with the epidemic better through reliance on logic and common sense.

Medical treatment recommended for buboes was to open them to let the infection out of the body. Muslim physician and poet Abu Khatima who practiced in Granada advised cutting only mature abscesses to make sure the patient does not bleed to death. In medieval times, surgery was sharply divided from internal medicine and counted as a menial job, and was not even taught at universities as part of medical curriculum. Surgeons on the other hand were more likely to have some training in medical theory. Barbersurgeons were trained through apprenticeship and had no training on theory. The role of apothecaries was to mix the medicines as directed by physicians.

Apart from the main categories, there were also non-registered unlicensed practitioners, such as midwives, who namely cared about the poor. Whilst surgery was left to surgeons, internal medicine in medieval times was often practiced by monks who were the only scholars with wide access to medical literature. Not all medieval physicians were university educated. Those who were consistently favored ancient teachings over experience. Humoralism, the predominant medieval medical theory, taught that the four bodily humors, black bile, yellow bile, blood, and phlegm, were affected by a person's diet, activity, and environment. One of the measures taken against plague by the populace were so called 'bowdy badges' – highly provocative items made of animal genitalia which were supposed to protect people against plague[33]. Old theories and medical teachings were helpless in face of the magnitude of devastation by the Black Death. Practitioners and surgeons, instead of blindly following official theories, became creative and relied on their own experience and judgment[34]. Matza in his thesis 'The sacred nature of secular medicine in the time of the Black Death' explains that medieval scholastic medicine was founded upon highly rationalized framework of nature and health, but simultaneously recognized divine agency as the logical cause and cure of human illness[35].

Relatively sudden disappearance of medical knowledge together with especially Jewish practitioners of medicine and surgery is linked to the concerted effort of newly asserted feudal rulers who were using Christian Church as a convenient oppressive method in order to keep the population in submission without having to use too much force which was sorely needed elsewhere for never ending crusades. Competing ideologies and philosophies were eliminated through burning of texts and expulsion of their proponents. Many Jewish physicians fled Europe because of anti-Semitic pogroms and took their Hebrew Bible and rabbinic scriptures with them. But expulsion of scholars would not be enough to stop people from thinking, no matter how limited their access to knowledge was.

---

[33] Gimbel, LM. 2012. "Bawdy Badges and the Black Death: Late Medieval Apotropaic Devices against the Spread of the Plague". A Thesis submitted to the Faculty of the College of Arts and Sciences of the University of Louisville.

[34] Vanneste, SF. 2010. "The Black Death and the Future of Medicine". Wayne State University.

[35] Matza, Louis. 2012. "The Sacred Nature of Secular Medicine in the Time of the Black Death". New Brunswick, New Jersey: Rutgers University.

Early medieval quest for heretics affected the most people who were not only intelligent, literate and well-read, but also outspoken and capable of formulating and communicating an independent judgment. People like that are extremely dangerous for any authoritarian regime because of their unpredictability, resilience to external pressures, intellectual independence, and constant quest for knowledge. This combination of traits in individuals, especially if combined with insensitivity to lack of approval by the community makes despots uncomfortable because of the potential for challenging the ruler's claim to power.

The psychology of medieval people was, however, very different. Rather than on physicians, they had to rely on religious explanation of the disaster which struck them. No treatment was offered to those who were affected by the disease; and the only advice provided to them was to turn to God. Authorities such as the Church, the ruler, and medicine, were failing in the face of Black Death, and people were largely left to their own devices. Some cities attempted to impose preventative measures, of which the most rational was a ring of fire which would protect certain areas from spreading of the disease.

Unity of State and Church did not allow the academic community to question religious dogmas. Medieval people were obsessed with their fate after death even before the plague, and during the outbreak even more so. Des Ormeaux pays lot of attention to the reaction of people to the pandemic, and the spread of terror and fear, and the desire to keep themselves alive. Paradoxically, milder outbreaks of plague in later years provoked more intense emotional reaction than the initial strike because certain psychological defenses apparently did not get activated and people were less likely to cope with the overwhelming presence of death through complete blocking of these memories. Ritual mass murders of Jews were common. As perceived culprits of the disease they were frequently used as scapegoats[36].

---

[36]   Des Ormeaux, AL. 2007. "The Black Death and Its Effect on Fourteen and Fifteen Century Art." Graduate Faculty of the Louisiana State University and Agricultural and Mechanical College.

The effects of authoritarian regimes on distribution of intellect in population are largely uncertain. From policy documents and historical records it is apparent that despots tend to systematically eliminate free thinkers and intellectual elite. How these measures affect the general population is subject to discussion because heritability (probability that a certain trait will be inherited) of psychometric, personal character, and intelligence traits is not only dependent on genetics but also on gene expression and environment. Manifestation of a trait tells us little about the genotype. While normal distribution of intelligence in population around the world is a factor studied by many researchers for its correlation to living standard and wealth, distribution of personality types around the globe is studied much less. There is no reason to assume that distribution of standardized personality types in population shall be more or less even. What the frequency does reveal is which types have been more successful throughout human existence. Myer-Briggs personality test describes four basic personality characteristics which depending on level of expression of the respective trait describe sixteen main personality types. The main measured characteristics are inclination toward introversion or extroversion, sensing or intuition, feeling or thinking, and judging vs. perception as characteristics of processing information and decision-making style. While distribution of some traits in population is more or less even, there is a striking disproportion in number of those who process information through sensing rather than intuition. Sensing types (ISFJ, ESFJ, and ISTJ) are also the most frequent personality types whilst N-J types (INFJ, ENFJ, INTJ, and ENTJ) are rarer. People who rely on their senses pay attention to physical reality and direct experience, whilst those who rely on intuition tend to systematically search for patterns and meaning of the information they are getting.

Intellectual capacity to correctly identify patterns may well be the cause why intuitive thinkers are consistently perceived by authoritarian regimes as threat. Current intelligence analysts employ sophisticated methods for identification of indicators of intent[37]. For dictators the distinction between capabilities and intentions is irrelevant; and mental capacity to process information in a structured manner counts as a well-defined threat regardless intent. In an authoritarian regime or oppressive theocracy an outspoken free thinker would be very unlikely to survive very long.

Medieval medicine was unable to do much for those who contracted plague; and only resorted to palliative care and spiritual assistance. The profession as whole completely resigned on combating the disease and succumbed to fatalism which engulfed Europe with the spread of plague. Astonishingly, fear of heresy was stronger than fear of plague; and scriptures which would have been helpful in combating the pandemic were not dug out from the archives and monasteries. Medicine of Dark Ages brought nothing to future generations of physicians in terms of knowledge. Did the millions of casualties of plague bring anything positive to medicine? The answer is – nothing at all.

---

[37]   Cragin, Kim, and Sara A Daly. 2004. "The Dynamic Terrorist Threat - An Assessment of Group Motivations and Capabilities in a Changing World." RAND Prepared for the United States Air Force.

III. MEDICAL OATHS

Medical profession is special because of the power a physician gains over human body due to his or her knowledge of its functions, and due to vast arsenal of means of affecting these bodily processes. Physicians are present at birth, and often also at the very moment of death. They often spend more time with the patient during his final moments than the family. Physicians are well aware of the power they have got over 'ordinary' people. The profession recognizes that there is a need for formal adherence to a set of values. This is achieved through an oath which is taken after graduation. Medical professionals all over the globe take an oath that they will fulfill the profession to the best of their ability and to the benefit of the patient. Unsurprisingly, the cradle of western civilization and continental legal system, ancient Greece, became the place where famous physician Hippocrates formulated the first oath for practitioners of this noble profession. This ancient oath, considered outdated by many, and only very rarely used without modifications, still serves as the most important ethical professional code in medicine. Hippocrates is rightly considered the father of modern western medicine. His teachings were based on empirical experience and careful observation. This principle is the core of modern medicine which is based on meticulous research and orientation towards the patient rather than interests of the doctor.

THE CODE OF HAMMURABI

The Code of Hammurabi consisted of 282 laws which were carved in stone around 1750 BC during the reign of Babylonian king Hammurabi (1792 – 1750 BC). The code covered wide range of matters from public to private: marriage and family relations; negligence; fraud; commercial contracts and fairness in commercial exchanges; duties of public officials; property and inheritance; crimes and punishments; techniques of legal procedures; protection for women, children, and slaves; protection of property; standard procedures for adjudicating disputes; debt relief for victims of food shortages and drought; and also guidelines for physicians and surgeons. Penalties imposed by the code varied according to the status of the victim which could be either patrician, plebeian, or a slave. Patricians, the highest class, were allowed to retaliate against the perpetrator following the spirit of the Old Testament – eye for eye and tooth for tooth. On the other hand, the lower classes were only entitled to monetary compensation. In regards to medicine, the code regulated malpractice and compensation for successful surgery or treatment, and penalties for any unsuccessful therapeutic procedures.[38] The Hammurabi code expected the physician or surgeon to treat only patients who could be cured, and imposed penalties for unsuccessful treatment attempts. The same applied to veterinarians. This code excluded any experimentation by default because any innovation inevitably would result in unsuccessful novel treatment attempts in some patients.

> 215. *If a surgeon has operated with the bronze lancet on a patrician for a serious injury, and has cured him, or has removed with a bronze lancet a cataract for a patrician, and has cured his eye, he shall take ten shekels of silver.*
>
> 216. *If it be a plebeian, he shall take five shekels of silver.*
>
> 217. *If it be a man's slave, the owner of the slave shall give two shekels of silver to the surgeon.*

---

[38] Sandlow, LJ. 2012. "Oaths, Codes, and Charters in Medicine over the Ages." *Hektoen International – A Journal of Medical Humanities* 3 (3).

218. If a surgeon has operated with the bronze lancet on a patrician for a serious injury, and has caused his death, or has removed a cataract for a patrician, with the bronze lancet, and has made him lose his eye, his hands shall be cut off.

219. If the surgeon has treated a serious injury of a plebeian's slave, with the bronze lancet, and has caused his death, he shall render slave for slave.

220. If he has removed a cataract with the bronze lancet, and made the slave lose his eye, he shall pay half his value.

221. If a surgeon has cured the limb of a patrician, or has doctored a diseased bowel, the patient shall pay five shekels of silver to the surgeon.

222. If he be a plebeian, he shall pay three shekels of silver.

223. If he be a man's slave, the owner of the slave shall give two shekels of silver to the doctor.

224. If a veterinary surgeon has treated an ox, or an ass, for a severe injury, and cured it, the owner of the ox, or the ass, shall pay the surgeon one-sixth of a shekel of silver, as his fee.

225. If he has treated an ox, or an ass, for a severe injury, and caused it to die, he shall pay one-quarter of its value to the owner of the ox, or the ass. [39] [40] [41]

---

[39] Hammurabi, and King LW (translator). "The Code of Hammurabi."

[40] Rev. Claude Hermann Walter Johns. 1910. "The Eleventh Edition of the Encyclopaedia Britannica."

[41] C. H. W. Johns. 2014. "The Avalon Project. Source: Babylonian and Assyrian Laws, Contracts and Letters, (1904), One of a Series Called the Library of Ancient Inscriptions, from a Facsimile Produced by The Legal Classics Library, Division of Gryphon Editions, New York in 1987."

THE VADAYA'S OATH

Hindu Physician's Oath (15th century BC) which was also known as the Vaidya's Oath extended physician's responsibilities to his lifestyle. Hindu physicians were not allowed to eat meat, drink alcoholic beverages, or commit adultery. Their conduct was supposed to be altruistic and free from earthly desires. This is probably also the only medical oath which expects the physician to treat all patients whom he meets on his errands including those who cannot afford to pay for his services.

HINDU PHYSICIAN'S OATH

You must put behind you desire, anger, greed, folly, pride, egotism, jealousy, harshness, calumny, falsehood, sloth and improper conduct.

With short-cut nails, ritually clean and clad in the orange garment, you must be pledged to truth, and full of reverence in addressing me...

If, however, you behave perfectly, while I profess false views, I shall be guilty of sin and my knowledge shall bear me no fruit.

(After having finished your studies) with your medicaments you shall assist Brahmins, venerable persons, poor people, women, ascetics, pious people seeking your assistance, widows and orphans and any one you meet on your errands, as if they were your own relatives. This will be right conduct.[42]

---

[42] Sandlow, LJ. 2012. "Oaths, Codes, and Charters in Medicine over the Ages." *Hektoen International – A Journal of Medical Humanities* 3 (3).

THE HIPPOCRATIC OATH

I swear by Apollo Physician and Asclepios and Hygeia and Panacea and all the gods and goddesses, making them my witnesses, that I will fulfill according to my ability and judgment this oath and this covenant: To hold him who has taught me this art as equal to my parents and to live my life in partnership with him, and if he is in need of money to give him a share of mine, and to regard his offspring as equal to my brothers in male lineage and to teach them this art — if they desire to learn it — without fee and covenant; to give a share of precepts and oral instruction and all the other learning to my sons and to the sons of him who has instructed me and to pupils who have signed the covenant and have taken an oath according to the medical law, but no one else.

The reference to polytheist Greek Gods was probably the reason why Hippocratic Oath[43] was forgotten during the Middle Ages and was only brought to light in early 1500s. Apollo, Asclepius, Hygeia, and Panacea, were replaced by a single God or anything what the concerned school held sacred. The selection of Gods reflects patrons of medical profession: Apollo was the healer and had power over plague; Asclepius, a son of Apollo rescued from his dead mother's womb, was instructed in the art of medicine by a centaur, and became recognized as the god of the medical art; Hygeia and Panacea, the daughters of Asclepius, were known as the goddess of good health and goddess of all cures. The reference to Gods is a reflection of respect to teachers and patrons rather than Supreme justice, which is as per the last paragraph taken care of by the patients and other medical professionals themselves. The profession was traditionally hereditary and handed down from father to son, a practice which is not unusual even today. This paragraph suggests that Medical Oath was in fact part of the law in ancient Greece, and was legally required for practitioners of medicine, something like a Pledge of Allegiance upon entering public service. These days, medical oath is still sworn during graduation ceremony at most medical schools, but does not have its

---

[43]   Hippocrates, and Ludwig Edelstein (Translation, interpretation). 1943. "From The Hippocratic Oath". Baltimore: Johns Hopkins Press.

legally binding meaning as it used to have. Access to information on the art of medicine, which can potentially cause harm if used inappropriately, was restricted to those who have taken the oath. In addition, the oath was taken and signed by students when commencing medical school and not upon completion of their studies. In ancient Greece, the meaning of medical oath was far less symbolic than it is now. It was a legal act. Today, medical profession is subject to regulations which to a certain degree replace the need for formal recognition of an ethical code. In 1928, only one fifth of medical schools in the United States let their students take an oath upon graduation. The situation changed dramatically after the Second World War as a result of the Nuremberg trials and introduction of the Nuremberg Code. Oath is now an integral part of graduation ceremonies at vast majority of schools all over the globe. Most schools use some type of modification to keep the oath up to date and consistent with modern values, but the spirit of Hippocrates's determination to have the benefit of the patient in mind at all times has not changed, not even after 2400 years.

> *I will apply dietetic measures for the benefit of the sick according to my ability and judgment; I will keep them from harm and injustice.*

The first remedy an ancient physician would consider is modification of patient's diet and lifestyle. Some authors reject the concept of Hippocratic medicine as paternalistic. It certainly does not seem to be the case with prescription of a diet because it is very hard to imagine a patient who would comply with a dietary regimen against his or her will. With lifestyle modification, trust between physician and patient is essential, just like the practitioner's authority.

> *I will neither give a deadly drug to anybody who asked for it, nor will I make a suggestion to this effect. Similarly I will not give to a woman an abortive remedy. In purity and holiness I will guard my life and my art.*

This part is often removed completely from the oath. Ban on euthanasia or assisted suicide is ingrained in the ancient code of medical ethics, just like the ban on abortions. The statement on not giving a deadly drug to "those who ask for it" does not necessarily mean the patient but anyone who might use it for other purpose than to benefit the patient. A pharmacist today would not be allowed to give a poison to whoever asks for it because this ancient principle present in the Hippocratic Oath was directly incorporated in law. Indian revised medical oath drafted by Dr. Rebello[44] in 2003 specifically mentions ban on administration of deadly drugs and harmful procedures:

> *I shall NOT prescribe lethal drugs, like anti-retrovirals, chemotherapy, or give electro-convulsive therapy to my patients.*

Modern Medical Oath available at the Indian Medical Association is not specific about administration of certain drugs and refers to the Indian Medical Council (Professional Conduct, Etiquette and Ethics) Regulations 2002[45].

> *I will not use the knife, not even on sufferers from stone, but will withdraw in favor of such men as are engaged in this work.*

When taken to a more abstract level, this principle is still valid today, as it reflects specialization in medicine and sharp division between internal medicine and surgery. General practitioners are only allowed to treat patients whose diseases do not require more specialized care, and are not supposed to perform surgical procedures they are not sufficiently trained in.

> *Whatever houses I may visit, I will come for the benefit of the sick, remaining free of all intentional injustice, of all mischief, and in particular of sexual relations with both female and male persons, be they free or slaves.*

Ban on sexual relationships with patients is still present in some cultures whilst left out from the Oath in others. In more general

---

[44]   Rebello, L. 2004. "Revised Doctors Oath. Independent Media Center India". Independent Media Center.

[45]   "Modern Oath." Indian Medical Association.

terms, this part refers to a dependent status of a patient on his physician, and the fact that this dependence should not be abused. The equivalent of ancient slaves would be people whose social status does not allow them full autonomy and therefore are more vulnerable to mistreatment or abuse. This statement can also be extended to persons whose health insurance status limits access to health care and who should not be exploited by the practitioner to benefit anyone else but the sick patient. It is easy to transfer this part of Hippocratic Oath to the current situation in exploitation of those with less means and limited legal protection in clinical trials especially in developing countries.

> *What I may see or hear in the course of the treatment or even outside of the treatment in regard to the life of men, which on no account one must spread abroad, I will keep to myself, holding such things shameful to be spoken about.*

Confidential relationship between the physician and the patient was of utmost importance to the ancient Greeks as they were well aware of the damage which inappropriate sharing of information can cause. Confidentiality applied not only to anything relating to the state of patient's health and treatment, but also to anything else what the practitioner learned due to the unique relationship with a patient. 'The life of men' represents any information the doctor gets due to his access to living quarters which remain private to all other people except for immediate family members. With this version of oath it would be very difficult to defend outsourcing of processing of sensitive medical information abroad. Within the medical fraternity, 59,095 doctors of Indian origin work abroad, primarily in the USA, UK, Canada, and Australia: 4.9 per cent of total number of doctors in the US and 10.9 per cent in Britain are of Indian descent[46]. Medicine has changed and data sharing across the globe became a widely accepted norm.

> *If I fulfill this oath and do not violate it, may it be granted to me to enjoy life and art, being honored with fame among all men for all time to come; if I transgress it and swear falsely, may the opposite of all this be my lot.*

---

[46]   Debroy, B. 2007. "A New Hippocratic Oath. The Indian Express"

Consequences of unethical conduct would be taken care of by very earthly means of suffering the life in infamy. This last sentence makes it clear that dealing with unethical conduct in medicine belongs to men and not to Gods, and that well performed medical art should be rewarded in terms of recognition and quality of life. In case of breach of the Hippocratic Oath the doctor shall be ostracized by the medical community and live in infamy. This principle evolved in formation of medical boards which are here to investigate professional misconduct and malpractice. This principle comes from the fact that only another doctor is qualified enough to judge appropriateness of treatment, and even when taken to non-medical institutions, expert opinion is always required by a jury.

The Hippocratic Oath is the oldest known and most widely used medical oath currently in use. It was reintroduced to Western medicine in 1508 at the University of Wittenberg in Germany; and eventually spread across the continent and beyond, with the wave of migrants from feudal Europe to America. The Oath was translated in English only in the beginning of 18th century. American Medical Association adopted its own medical oath in 1847, more than half a century after introduction of Thomas Percival's oath in Europe.

In 1928, only about one fifth of American medical graduates took some form of medical oath. This dramatically changed after the Second World War as a result of the Nuremberg Trials and introduction of the Declaration of Geneva in 1948. This does not mean that a standardized medical oath is sworn by medical students across the country or even across the globe; in fact the opposite is true. While about 50% American schools opted for the Hippocratic Oath with some modifications and modernization, others have chosen a different oath such as the Declaration of Geneva which was drafted in 1948, or the Lasagna Oath from 1964, or composed their own oaths[47].

---

[47]   Hulkover R. 2010. "The History of the Hippocratic Oath: Outdated, Inauthentic, and Yet Still Relevant." *The Einstein Journal of Biology and Medicine*, 41−44.

Some sort of oath is required by medical schools either upon entering the school or upon leaving. The number of students swearing an oath equals 100% in many countries including the USA, Russia, China, the Netherlands, Singapore, or Poland[48]. Hippocrates still appeals to the medical community because his texts contain vast amount of medical information and display then revolutionary attitude towards the practice of medicine: attitude which emphasizes nature over philosophy and observation over theoretical dogmas and reasoning; and which puts patient's interest before that of the physician. These principles were abandoned for long periods of time: first in the Middle Ages as the consequence of loss of autonomy among peoples of feudal Europe; and later, during the ascent of totalitarian regimes – Nazi, Fascist, and Communist alike – as a consequence of precisely the same – loss of autonomy.

There are some academics, namely Engelhardt and Veatch who believe that taking an oath in medical profession is inappropriate. Whilst Engelhardt rejects medical oath on the basis of absence of universal values and pluralist understanding of morality in contemporary culture, Veatch finds the Hippocratic Oath too empowering for the physician. In his opinion, the phrase "according to my ability and judgment" encourages paternalism[49]. This approach is very understandable considering the fact that medicine was a secret art and no commoner would have had any chance of knowing whether the physician is doing the right thing or not. The profession relied on the power of good or bad reputation and the idea that good physicians would not tolerate bad ones in their ranks.

---

[48] Radomyski, Mateusz. 2011. "Medical Oaths: When Religion and Ethics Collide." *Amsterdam Law Forum* 3 (1): 68–80.

[49] Ibid.

THE OATH OF ASAPH & YOHANAN

This Hebrew oath was taught to students of Asaph and Yohanan (6th century AD), and included ethical standards regarding the sanctity of life (euthanasia and abortion), bribery, and doctor-patient confidentiality. The oath also urges the physician to be compassionate with the poor and the needy. The ban on abortions is only limited to women who got pregnant as a result of intimate relationship outside wedlock and not to those who were married and got pregnant with their own husband. This seems counter-intuitive, as the prospects of illegitimate children always had been very grim. On the other hand, rivalries among siblings certainly created lot of pressure on a woman not to have any more children because of greater number of youngsters potentially claiming inheritance and dividing land. The oath also refers to practices which were apparently common at that time and which are still in use today in some cultures where arranged marriages are practiced, and compliance of both marriage partners has to be ensured. Techniques which would break emotional bonds where these are undesired, or facilitate formation of relationships which would not spontaneously occur were condemned as sorcery or witchcraft and shall never be performed by a physician. The same ban applied to any efforts to deprive a woman of her beauty.

The Asaph & Yohanan oath fully separated activities performed by priests (worship) with regards to healing powers and those performed by physicians. Those who seek help of charlatans shall be informed that demons and spirits of the dead have no power over their own corpses and therefore cannot be expected to have the ability to provide any assistance to the living. The final statement reminds the physicians to respect God as the only power which can heal; and that even the most brilliant intellect should not dare to challenge God or play God. In the difference from Hippocrates, who relied on earthly justice with regards to medical malpractice, Asaph and Yohanan referred to God as the one who sees all and knows all, and physicians shall always take into consideration this when engaging in any sort of mischief.

Do not attempt to kill any soul by means of a portion of herbs; do not make a woman [who is] pregnant [as a result of] of whoring take a drink with a view to causing abortion,

Do not covet beauty of form in women with a view to fornicating with them; do not divulge the secret of a man, who has trusted you,

Do not take any reward [which may be offered in order to induce you] to destroy and to ruin,

Do not harden your heart [and turn it away] from pitying the poor and healing the needy; do not say of [what is] good; it is bad, nor of [what is] bad; it is good,

Do not adopt the ways of the sorcerers using [as they do] charms, augury, and sorcery in order to separate a man from the wife of his bosom or a woman from the companion of her youth,

You shall not covet any wealth or reward [which may be offered in order to induce you] to help in a lustful desire,

You shall not seek help in any idolatrous [worship] so as to heal through [a recourse to idols], and you shall not heal with anything [pertaining] to their worship,

But on the contrary detest and abhor and hate all those who worship them, put their trust in them, and give assurance [referring] to them,

For they are all naught, useless, for they are nothing, demons, spirits of the dead; they cannot help their own corpses, how then could they help those who live?

Now [then] put your trust in the Lord, your God, [who is] a true God, a living God; for [it is] He who kills and makes alive, who wounds and heals, who teaches men knowledge and also to profit,

Who wounds with justice and righteousness, and who heals with pity and compassion,

No designs of [His] sagacity are beyond His [power] and nothing is hidden from His eyes.[50]

---

[50]   Sandlow, LJ. 2012. "Oaths, Codes, and Charters in Medicine over the Ages." *Hektoen International – A Journal of Medical Humanities* 3 (3).

THE OATH OF SUN SIMIAO

Sun Simiao (581-682 CE) was known as the Chinese Hippocrates or China's King of Medicine. He was the famous doctor of the Sui and Tang Dynasty. The Sui Dynasty was founded by Yang Chien, a general who first conquered Northern Chou, and then through campaigns to the south he reunified China. First time in four centuries China was under unified centralized administrative power. The north became badly decimated as a result of these wars and Yang Chien had to establish communication and logistical channels which would allow shipping of goods from south to north. Ambitious projects, extensive defensive border works, and continuing invasions abroad to Korea and current North Vietnam exhausted the country and caused lot of suffering among the local population.[51]

Status, wealth or age, attractiveness, or nationality of the patient should not sway the physician's determination to provide necessary assistance. All should be treated with the utmost care. In spirit, this oath closely resembles the ideas of compassion with enemy sick and wounded which were later codified in the Geneva Conventions. Providing medical care to the subdued by physicians who belonged to the invading force was part of psychological operations relating to conquest of territory.

> 'A Great Physician should not pay attention to status, wealth or age; neither should he question whether the particular person is attractive or unattractive, whether he is an enemy or friend, whether he is a Chinese or a foreigner, or finally, whether he is uneducated or educated. He should meet everyone on equal grounds. He should always act as if he were thinking of his close relatives.'[52]

---

[51]   Sawyer, RD. *The TAO of Deception. Unorthodox Warfare in Historic and Modern China. Chapter Sui and T'ang Conflicts, Basic Books, 2007; pp 189 – 211.*

[52]   Sandlow LJ: Oaths, codes, and charters in medicine over the ages. Hektoen International – A Journal of Medical Humanities, 2012; Volume 3, Issue 3.

THE OATH AND THE PRAYER OF MAIMONIDES

The Oath of Maimonides is named after a great Hebrew physician Moses Maimonides, also known as Rabbi Moshe Ben Maimon, RaMBaM, or Abu 'Imran Musa ben Maimun ibn 'Abd Allah, the author of ten works on medicine and Jewish law, an important opponent of witchcraft and supporter of rational measures in medicine, including clean surgical technique. The Oath emphasizes philanthropy and truth, and continuous learning and permanent status of adjustment of medical practice to expanding knowledge about diseases and their treatment.

In context of other works of that time, Maimonides' philosophy of science was breathtakingly rational. It is no coincidence that his works inspired many ethicist philosophers of later time, especially renaissance Jewish philosopher Baruch Spinoza (1632 – 1677) who was inspired by Maimonides' view of human eudaimonia. Spinoza argued that the mind's intellectual love of God is our understanding of the universe, our virtue, our happiness, our well-being and our 'salvation'. It is also our freedom and autonomy.[53]

There is no doubt that autonomy of patients in the era between Maimonides and Spinoza, in other words between the First and Second Renaissance, was severely limited, not only with respect to their religious beliefs, but also all other means of self-determination. Loss of autonomy and personal freedom, limitation on choices and individual precautions, were part of the circumstances which made the 1348 plague pandemic so deadly. Medieval Christian society had no capacity to tackle the pandemic because of absence of 'truth' in their theories.

---

[53]   Steven Nadler. "Baruch Spinoza." *Stanford Encyclopedia of Philosophy.* Stanford University. 2001, rev. 2013.

The Oath of Maimonides

The eternal providence has appointed me to watch over the life and health of Thy creatures. May the love for my art actuate me at all time; may neither avarice nor miserliness, nor thirst for glory or for a great reputation engage my mind; for the enemies of truth and philanthropy could easily deceive me and make me forgetful of my lofty aim of doing good to Thy children. May I never see in the patient anything but a fellow creature in pain. Grant me the strength, time and opportunity always to correct what I have acquired, always to extend its domain; for knowledge is immense and the spirit of man can extend indefinitely to enrich itself daily with new requirements. Today he can discover his errors of yesterday and tomorrow he can obtain a new light on what he thinks himself sure of today. Oh, God, Thou has appointed me to watch over the life and death of Thy creatures; here am I ready for my vocation and now I turn unto my calling.[54]

The Prayer of Maimonides

The 'Daily Prayer Of A Physician' is attributed to Maimonides, but was probably written by Marcus Herz, a German physician, pupil of Immanual Kant, and physician to Moses Mendelssohn. It first appeared in print in about 1793. The fact that these 12th century texts were rediscovered in 17th and 18th century and extensively studied by the best philosophers of those days shows how modern these ideas were for the Enlightenment movement.

Almighty God, Thou has created the human body with infinite wisdom. Ten thousand times ten thousand organs hast Thou combined in it that act unceasingly and harmoniously to preserve the whole in all its beauty the body which is the envelope of the immortal soul.

They are ever acting in perfect order, agreement and accord. Yet, when the frailty of matter or the unbridling of passions deranges this order or interrupts this accord, then forces clash and the body

---

[54]   Moses Maimonides. 1917. "The Oath of Maimonides and The Prayer of Maimonides." *Bulletin of the Johns Hopkins Hospital* 28: 260–61.

crumbles into the primal dust from which it came. Thou sendest to man diseases as beneficent messengers to foretell approaching danger and to urge him to avert it.

Thou has blest Thine earth, Thy rivers and Thy mountains with healing substances; they enable Thy creatures to alleviate their sufferings and to heal their illnesses. Thou hast endowed man with the wisdom to relieve the suffering of his brother, to recognize his disorders, to extract the healing substances, to discover their powers and to prepare and to apply them to suit every ill.

In Thine Eternal Providence Thou hast chosen me to watch over the life and health of Thy creatures. I am now about to apply myself to the duties of my profession.

Support me, Almighty God, in these great labors that they may benefit mankind, for without Thy help not even the least thing will succeed.

Inspire me with love for my art and for Thy creatures. Do not allow thirst for profit, ambition for renown and admiration, to interfere with my profession, for these are the enemies of truth and of love for mankind and they can lead astray in the great task of attending to the welfare of Thy creatures.

Preserve the strength of my body and of my soul that they ever be ready to cheerfully help and support rich and poor, good and bad, enemy as well as friend. In the sufferer let me see only the human being.

Illumine my mind that it recognize what presents itself and that it may comprehend what is absent or hidden.

Let it not fail to see what is visible, but do not permit it to arrogate to itself the power to see what cannot be seen, for delicate and indefinite are the bounds of the great art of caring for the lives and health of Thy creatures.

Let me never be absent- minded.

May no strange thoughts divert my attention at the bedside of the sick, or disturb my mind in its silent labors, for great and sacred are the thoughtful deliberations required to preserve the lives and health of Thy creatures.

Grant that my patients have confidence in me and my art and follow my directions and my counsel. Remove from their midst all charlatans and the whole host of officious relatives and know-all nurses, cruel people who arrogantly frustrate the wisest purposes of our art and often lead Thy creatures to their death.

Should those who are wiser than I wish to improve and instruct me, let my soul gratefully follow their guidance; for vast is the extent of our art.

Should conceited fools, however, censure me, then let love for my profession steel me against them, so that I remain steadfast without regard for age, for reputation, or for honor, because surrender would bring to Thy creatures sickness and death.

Imbue my soul with gentleness and calmness when older colleagues, proud of their age, wish to displace me or to scorn me or disdainfully to teach me.

May even this be of advantage to me, for they know many things of which I am ignorant, but let not their arrogance give me pain. For they are old and old age is not master of the passions.

I also hope to attain old age upon this earth, before Thee, Almighty God!

Let me be contented in everything except in the great science of my profession.

Never allow the thought to arise in me that I have attained to sufficient knowledge, but vouchsafe to me the strength, the leisure and the ambition ever to extend my knowledge. For art is great, but the mind of man is ever expanding.

Almighty God! Thou hast chosen me in Thy mercy to watch over the life and death of Thy creatures.

I now apply myself to my profession. Support me in this great task so that it may benefit mankind, for without Thy help not even the least thing will succeed.[55]

---

[55]   Moses Maimonides. 1917. "The Oath of Maimonides and The Prayer of Maimonides." *Bulletin of the Johns Hopkins Hospital* 28: 260–61.

THE JOURNEY OF A PHYSICIAN – THE OATH OF THE SCHOOL OF ENJUIN

Traditional Japanese medical ethics stems from Buddhist, Confucian, and Shinto tradition. The same combination of Buddhism, Shinto, and Confucianism, unique to Japan, fundamentally influenced Japanese martial arts. In both arts, martial and medical, detailed knowledge of human body and its function and limits is essential.

The Oath of the School of Enjuin

Each person should follow the path designated by Heaven.

You should always be kind to people. You should always be devoted to loving people.

The teaching of Medicine should be restricted to selected persons.

You should not tell others what you are taught, regarding treatments without permission

You should not establish association with doctors who do not belong to this school. All the successors and descendants of the disciples of this school shall follow the teachers' ways.

If any disciples cease the practice of Medicine, or, if successors are not found at the death of the disciple, all the medical books of this school should be returned to the School of Enjuin.

You should not kill living creatures, nor should you admire hunting or fishing.

In our school, teaching about poisons is prohibited; neither should you receive instructions about poisons from other physicians. Moreover, you should not give abortive to the people.

You should rescue even such patients as you dislike or hate. You should do virtuous acts, but in such a way that they do not become known to people. To do good deeds secretly is a mark of virtue.

You should not exhibit avarice and you must not strain to become famous. You should not rebuke or reprove a patient, even if he does not present you with money or goods in gratitude.

You should be delighted if, after treating a patient without success, the patient receives medicine from another physician, and is cured.

You should not speak ill of other physicians.

You should not tell what you have learned from the time you enter a woman's room, and, moreover, you should not have obscene or immoral feelings when examining a woman.

Proper or not, you should not tell others what you have learned in lectures, or what you have learned about prescribing medicine.

You should not like undue extravagance. If you like such living, your avarice will increase, and you will lose the ability to be kind to others.

If you do not keep the rules and regulations of this school, then you will be cancelled as a disciple. In more severe cases, the punishment will be greater.[56]

The Bushido Code

There was probably no other culture except for Korea and China, where martial arts had the same tradition as in Japan, where the art of medicine would be so closely tied to the art of hand-to-hand combat. Both codes, Bushido and Enjuin School (15th century AD), were written during the two-hundred-fifty years peacetime period under the rule of Hideyoshi when many Samurais were leading secret arts schools as part of their searching for purpose in life at time of long peace. The title samurai was originally reserved for men of noble birth who had training in archery, unarmed combat techniques, and sword techniques who were assigned to guard members of the Imperial Court. Professional Japanese warriors

---

[56]   Reich WT. 1995. "The Oath of the School of Enjuin." *Encyclopedia of Bioethics.* Revised Edition Vol 5. New York: Simon & Schuster MacMillan.

Samurais knew function and limits of human body better than any western physician of that time because of the very fact of extreme training which was passed down from generation to generation as the most closely guarded secret. Japanese code of medical ethics which is known as 'The 17 rules of Enjuin' was developed for students of Ri-shu school in sixteenth century. Just like martial arts, medicine was kept away from all outsiders. In principles, The 17 rules of Enjuin resemble the Bushido code, known as the journey of Samurai. Buddhist texts stress the importance of moral virtues called perfections including generosity, tolerance, truthfulness, and vigor, and avoid the concept of ethical behavior altogether. Some Buddhist teachers such as for example Thomas Kasulis argue that Buddhism establishes a virtue ethics with a central focus on a moral person rather than moral act.

Many Buddhists accept the Noble Eightfold Path and the basic Buddhist precepts as simple, straightforward, practical guides to leading a virtuous life. Buddhist moral code is based on consequentiality and acceptance of responsibility for willful acts, no matter whether good or evil. Bushido, the Samurai code of conduct, was a set of Seven Virtues that the Samurai of Japan and ancient warriors of China and Korea had to live and die by. As per modern interpretation taught in various martial art schools, '**Gi**' stands for the right decision, rectitude, fairness, and rightful use of authority; '**Yu**' for bravery, heroism, courage, and ability to face danger without hesitation and without loss of self-esteem; '**Jin**' for benevolence, kindness, and ability to be charitable; '**Rel**' for the right action, '**Rei**' or Reishiki etiquette as preservation of courtesy, respect and politeness; '**Makoto**' for sincerity, truthfulness, honesty, accuracy, and precision; '**Melyo**' for honor, adherence to principles which are right, and glory without ego; and '**Chugo**' for loyalty, devotion to ones lord and obedience to teacher, and faithfulness to family, friends, country, and ideals. In addition to the Seven Virtues mentioned in the Bushido Code martial arts schools emphasized filial piety in the sense of respect to ones ancestors; building of character and self-control; and wisdom, resourcefulness, and wit.

In 1185 Minamoto no Yoritomo, a daimyo (warlord) of the eastern provinces who traced his lineage back to the imperial family, established the nation's first military government (1185-1867) which lasted nearly seven centuries. The only power which ever tried to invade Japan – and failed – was Kublai Khan's Mongol Empire. Kublai Khan, grandson of Chingiz Khan, and founder of the Mongol Yuan dynasty which ruled over most of eastern Asia until 1368, attempted to invade Japan twice during his reign: first time in 1274 and the second time seven years later, in 1281. The Mongols landed at Hakata Bay, the Kyushu Island, and met fierce resistance of the Samurais under the leadership of Kikuchi Takefusa and Takezaki Suenaga. Retreating Mongols split in two groups and headed for Sohara and Tsukahara, whilst Samurais left the battlefield, having achieved victory for which they could claim reward from their masters. Takazaki Suanaga's forces then attacked the Mongols at Tsukahara and forced them to withdraw. After an extended battle at Sohara, Samurais retreated to ancient fortress Mizuki and unattended Mongols set afire several shrines on the coast before leaving Japan the next day, leaving behind their ponies. For Japanese horse breeds this was a very welcome refreshment of otherwise very limited gene pool. All three main types, mountain pony Kiso, wild pony Kigoshima from Kyushu, and grasslands pony Hokkaido have only about 132 cm withers height, and this unexpected import of Mongol war horses made a difference.

In 1275, Japanese defenders started building walls behind the beaches which paid off during the second Mongol invasion attempt.[57] Mongol forces could not land because of the fortifications and had to stay off shore, gradually depleting their water supplies. Samurais were getting ready for a fight and as a part of these preparations they prayed extensively. Natural forces intervened and the Mongol fleet waiting for their opportunity was destroyed by a hundred years storm. The Japanese called this fortunate natural phenomenon a Divine Wind, 'Kamikaze'. Although the invasions of Japan by Mongols failed, Japan was not heading for a period of peace. In 1467 the national military government collapsed and the infamous Age of Wars begun. The term Samurai changed its meaning and could represent almost

---

[57]   Bowdoin College. "Bowdoin: The Mongol Invasions of Japan 1274 – 1281. " *Bowdoin: Asian Studies.*

anyone from armed government officials, peacekeeping officers, and professional soldiers to street thugs. The power shifted from Imperial government to independent rulers who called themselves Daimyo. Samurais frequently had to switch sides when the battles were not developing the way they expected or when their master perished in battle. In the difference from most of the population, Samurais were highly literate and kept meticulous records of details of each conflict and especially their own injuries to be able to seek compensation. To prove their invaluable service, they used to cut off head of their enemies for which they would be paid. This practice led to establishment of head-viewing committees which forensically examined the fetched heads in order to find out whether it was really cut off a living or freshly killed warrior or collected from a dead body. In such a case the Samurai naturally would not get paid but would be punished for cheating. Sixteenth century was the most fruitful time for Samurais.

The struggle between Daimyos provided plentiful opportunities for those who desired to improve their social standing through military service. Two extraordinary Daimyos of this time were Uesuga Kenshin and Takeda Shingen, contemporaries, neighbors, and rivals. When they finally had the opportunity to dispose of one another, let their opponent go out of chivalry. Until 1400's military training in Japan was largely informal but this was about to change with fast development of kendo techniques starting late 15th century when more formal mentoring of future Samurais started in warrior schools. Renowned swordsman Tsukuhara Bokuden, after many years of war fighting during which he took part in more than 30 major battles, became tired of young Samurais who were constantly trying to challenge him to earn fame, and developed non-lethal unarmed techniques which he taught others. As he grew older, he adopted more peaceful attitude which mainly involved the art of winning without fighting. Many Samurais of these days had no noble lineage and the actions which brought them to the top of medieval social ladder were less than honorable and involved lot of bloodshed. In 1568, ambitious Daimyo Oda Nobunaga conceived an idea that Japan would be better off united and started acting on his ideas through marriages arranged between powerful families, and intimidation and fierce fighting of those who did not want to join. Nobunaga utilized to the full firearms which first reached

Japan in 1543 due to Portuguese merchants and by mastering this new technique he managed to stop armies many times his size. Nobunaga did not live long enough to see Japan united and died by the hand of an assassin. His successor Toyotomi Hideyoshi got to power due to a cunning trick. Hideyoshi tracked down Nobunaga's assassin and killed him what gave him gratitude of Nobunaga's heir for active revenge whilst Hideyoshi seized power.

The process of unification of Japan continued through combination of cunning political maneuvering and ruthless military might. When in 1590 finally all local rulers submitted to Hideyoshi's rule, Japan's military culture suddenly came to an end. Hideyoshi implemented gun control and ordered all swords to be melted down to build statues of Buddha which symbolized lasting peace. Freezing of social mobility followed immediately after disposal of any potential armed resistance. Classes of feudal society formed distinct borders between them. Samurais, the only class which was allowed to bear arms, were set apart from the rest of society. They had the right to have two swords, a long and a short one, but had to give up any ties to land. Commoners, the farmers, the artisans, and the merchants, were allowed to own land but were not allowed to bear arms.

Although the imperial family had almost no political power, Hideyoshi could not reach the top rank of Shogun because of his humble origins. He eventually died in his bed aged 62 in 1598 leaving his 5-year old son as an heir protected by an army of loyalists. In October 1600 Tokugawa's army defeated Hideyoshi's loyalists by persuading many of them to switch sides. In 1603 Tokugawa submitted a false claim that he is related to the Imperial family. Nobody challenged his claim and his title was approved. Japan entered period of two-and-half centuries of peace which was enforced by an iron hand.

Local rules were so committed to peace that they frequently exchanged relatives to prove determination not to fight. These 'family exchanges' more resembled hostage taking and became inspiration for the tradition of 'keeping of guests' at the expense of

Emperor during the World War Two. Most Japanese could not travel abroad and their domestic traveling was under strict control to prevent accumulation of hostile forces. To keep the isolation complete only very few foreigners were let in.

The Code of a Samurai and the Code of the School of Enjuin were written during the period of unusually long peace in Japanese history. Samurais as a class did not disappear but had nothing to do because there were no wars. Their role in society partially vanished and partially morphed. They could not own land and did not engage in trade either, living off stipends paid by their landlords and governors should their services ever be needed. If they wanted to sit idle they easily could have, but they did not. First of all, Samurais were traditionally hyperactive and also exceptionally literate compared to other segments of Japanese society. In this sense they felt responsible for maintaining their unique status and this included spiritual leadership. Some Samurais pursued careers in public administration; others became poets and artists or masters of ikebana or drama. Martial arts schools blossomed. Training schools differed in style but one trend was shared by all: they became much more ritualized and formalized. Styles such as Kendo and Iaido taught sword techniques whilst others specialized in unarmed close combat. Some, like karate, used powerful punches and kicks, whilst other styles, like aikido, taught to utilize energy of the opponent to achieve victory.

The period of tranquility ended in 1853 when U.S. warships disturbed this peace by asking Japan for permission to build a port for whaling. Japanese warriors suddenly faced modern navy with which they had no chance of competing should the visiting power be hostile. In 1867 the Last Shogun Tokugama Keiki relinquished power to young Emperor Meiji who led the country until 1912, enforcing rapid industrialization. Public wearing of swords was outlawed and the warrior class was abolished, something what Hideyoshi never fully achieved: a sword-less samurai.[58]

---

[58] Brett McKay, and Kate McKay. 2008. "The Bushido Code: The Eight Virtues of the Samurai."

The warrior code was used as inspiration for the entire nation and during the Second World War became the cause of complete disregard of Japanese soldiers for their own lives. They would rather die than surrender, and expected the same way of thinking from opposing forces. Opposing forces on the other hand expected way of thinking they were familiar with. The question is what happened to Japanese doctors during the Second World War that they felt free to conduct horrendous experiments on Allied prisoners of war when they had indeed Medical Code of Ethics and were party to the Geneva Conventions. The answer is easy. The Oath of School of Enjun did not apply to prisoners of war. The Samurai Code did.

After the attack on Pearl Harbor[59], Japanese imperial forces advanced through the Pacific Islands toward Australia. Their attempted invasion of Port Moresby was thwarted in May 1942 by Admiral Nimitz's fleet which clashed with Admiral Shigeyohi in the Coral Sea. The Americans suffered heavy losses including carrier Lexington. Admiral Chester Nimitz, key American naval commander in the Pacific Theater of operations, was directly involved in both planning and execution of the most important battles against the Japanese during WW2[60].

The first major shift in balance of power came with the Battle of Midway in June 1942 when all four heavy carriers of Yamamoto's fleet were sunk[61]. In July 1942, the Japanese seized Guadalcanal. The battle over this island took half a year and inspired among others famous Terrence Malik's film 'The Thin Red Line'[62]. The Americans finally took control of the island in February 1943. The battles of the Gilbert Islands Tarawa and Makin in November 1943 alone claimed 3,000 American casualties.

---

[59] Department of Defense. "Overview of the Pearl Harbor Attack, December 7, 1941." *Naval History and Heritage Command.*

[60] Jeremy Black. 2008. *Great Military Leaders and Their Campaigns: Admiral Nimitz, Successful Commander of American Naval Forces against Japan, Pp 274-9.* London: Thames & Hudson.

[61] *National Geographic's Battle for Midway.* 2001. National Geographic Videos.

[62] Terrence Mallick. 1998. *The Thin Red Line.*

In 1944, during the Mariana Islands and Palau campaigns, the determination of Japanese forces was shown in full light. Almost entire garrison of 27,000 men based at vital bomber base in Saipan, died in an attack and refused to surrender. In October 1944, in Operation Sho, the Japanese threatened the landing fleet during the American invasion of the Philippines, but did not succeed. The invasions of Iwo Jima in February 1945 and Okinawa from March to June 1945 were meant to provide air bases for the planned invasion of Japan[63]. The nuclear attacks on Hiroshima and Nagasaki on August 6 and 9, 1945, finally forced Japan to surrender[64].

In mid-August 1945, the Imperial Japanese Army was spread all over the Pacific. The estimated strength of the Japanese Army was more than 6,6 million troops: 1,620,516 in the USSR and Northern part of Korea; 595,418 in South Korea; 1,105,837 in Manchuria; 1,501,260 in China; 19,222 in Hong Kong; 479,313 in Formosa; 69,374 in Ryukyus; 62,389 in Bonim islands; 32,037 in Northern part of French Indochina; 710,727 in South East Asia (Burma, Thailand, Southern part of French Indochina, and Malaya); 132,917 in the Philippines; 130,906 in the Marianas and Marshall Islands; 15,590 in Borneo, Netherland Indies, and Western part of New Guinea; and 138,680 in Eastern part of New Guinea, Bismarck Archipelago, and Solomon Islands.[65]

The total number of U.S. and British military personnel captured by all Axis forces was about 367.000 persons. Among the 235.000 U.S. and British prisoners of war captured by Germans and Italians, the death toll was about 4%. Of 132.000 POWs who fell in the

---

[63]   Jeremy Black. 2008. *Great Military Leaders and Their Campaigns: Admiral Nimitz, Successful Commander of American Naval Forces against Japan, Pp 274-9.* London: Thames & Hudson.

[64]   "U.S. Strategic Bombing Survey. The Effects of the Atomic Bombings of Hiroshima and Nagasaki. Chairman's Office, June 19, 1946." *The Truman Library.* Project Whistlestop.

[65]   James McNaughton. 2006. *Nisei Linguists: Japanese Americans in the Military Intelligence Service during World War II. Map 15, Pp 388-389.* Department of the Army, Washington D.C.

hands of the Japanese, 27% died. Main causes of death were starvation and malnutrition, disease and lack of health care. Many died on board of hell ships during transport to Japan, or succumbed to exhaustion during forced marches and slave labor. Many died of consequences of beating. Some were randomly killed by guards. Hundreds of thousands of Allied POWs were forced to build Thai-Burma railway.[66] Mistreatment of POWs and withdrawal of aid provided by the Allies raised serious concerns during the war. Irrefutable evidence that Allied POWs were used as subjects for medical experiments or for biological and chemical warfare research is hard to come by.

Unit 731 was not the only unit where the Japanese tested biological and chemical warfare; there were also units 1855 in Beijing, 1644 in Nanjing (Tama Unit), and 1688 in Canton. Whether the Japanese intended to use biological warfare against the USA or not will never be known for certain, although the development of air balloons which were sent to over the U.S. mainland using meteorological phenomenon jet-stream, and the fact that these weapons were tested in China, suggest that this was more than only a theoretical possibility.[67]

Most research subjects were Chinese, Russian, and Mongolian nationals. General MacArthur obtained intelligence about Japanese biological and chemical warfare research in Manchuria already in mid-1944 from the Allied Translator and Interpreter Section (ATIS) including information on the so-called 'bacillus bomb' and research report on medical war crimes, including the incident at Kyushu Imperial University where American pilots were dissected out of 'curiosity'. In 1948, 30 doctors were charged with vivisection, wrongful removal of bodily parts, and cannibalism; 23 were

---

[66] Daqing Yang. 2006. "Documentary Evidence and Studies of Japanese War Crimes: An Interim Assessment." In *Researching Japanese War Crimes Records: Introductory Essays*, 21–56. National Archives and Records Administration for the Nazi War Crimes and Japanese Imperial Government Records Interagency Working Group.

[67] Ibid, pp 21-56.

convicted.[68]

Japanese General Ishii Shiro was the man responsible for Unit 731 laboratories at Pingfan near Harbin, Manchuria. At least 3,000 were killed in experiments at the Unit 731 biological weapons facility, reportedly including gunned down Allied airmen. Experiments conducted at Unit 731 included vivisections, freezing and amputations of limbs to study spread of gangrene and blood loss, removal of organs such as parts of brain, lungs, and liver to study disease, and tests of explosives on human body. In total, approximately 200,000 were killed in field tests of biological weapons in a project code-named 'Maruta'.

After the surrender of Japan, General Ishii Shiro ordered to kill all the experimental subjects by potassium cyanide in their food, or gas them to death with mustard gas or phosgene. Their bodies were stuffed in incinerators and dumped in a pit in the courtyard and burned. Ishii Shiro ordered his staff and family to commit suicide and even issued poison for them all. Hardly any of these people followed the order; and approximately 2,000 of them including Ishii fled the camp instead. On departure, they released thousands of bubonic plague-infected rats, what directly led to the death of another 20,000 to 30,000 Chinese. Some of the scientists involved were later tried in the Tokyo War Crimes Tribunal and the Khabarovsk War Crime Trial; most escaped to the West and succeeded in business, academia, politics, and medicine. According to the Unit 731 Testimony, General Douglass Mac Arthur secretly granted immunity to the physicians of Unit 731 in exchange for providing America with their research on chemical and biological warfare.

According to the 2002 International Symposium on the Crimes of Bacteriological Warfare, the number of people killed by the

---

[68]   E Drea, G Bradsher, R Hanyok, J Lide, M Petersen, and D Yang. 2006. "Nazi War Crimes and Japanese Imperial Government Records Interagency Working Group." In *Researching Japanese War Crimes Records Introductory Essays.*, 79–110. Japanese War Crimes Records at the National Archives: Research Starting Points. Washington D.C.

Imperial Japanese Army germ warfare and human experiments is about 580,000, most of it Chinese civilians killed by cholera, typhoid, anthrax, bubonic plague, and tularemia. Japanese law does not define those convicted in the post-1945 trials as criminals, despite the fact that Japan's governments have accepted the judgments made in the trials as spelled out in the Treaty of San Francisco (1952). In 1993, U.S. Defense Secretary William Perry finally promised to declassify records of WW2 experiments. The result of this effort is an impressive study 'Japanese War Crimes Records Introductory Essays' which was published in 2006[69].

Unit 731 was not the only one which conducted vivisections on prisoners. Wartime surgeon Dr Ken Yuasa in his testimonies described these practices also in Imperial Japanese Army hospital in Luan (now Changzhi) in Shanxi Province in China in February 1942. Yuasa stated that his nationalist indoctrination and schooling was stronger than his conscience; and that he believed that front-line soldiers committed much worse atrocities than they did in the hospital. It took only six weeks to become a coldblooded vivisectionist. After the War, Yuasa practiced medicine until 84 years of age.[70]

Complete loss of any sense of conscience is obvious from meticulous record-keeping and scientific evaluation of 'logs'. Ishii himself patented over 200 discoveries. After the war, U.S. representatives refused to deal with the atrocities and force the Japanese to face trial. Opposite is true; they were granted impunity in exchange for data and cooperation. Of 200 surviving POWs, only one was allowed to testify in Congress as late as in 1982.[71] Many doctors who participated in Japanese Biological Warfare Research

---

[69]   Drea E, Bradsher G, Hanyok R, Lide J, Petersen M, Yang D: Researching Japanese War Crimes Records Introductory Essays. Nazi War Crimes and Japanese Imperial Government Records Interagency Working Group. Washington D.C. 2006.

[70]   Jun Hongo. 2007. "Vivisectionist Recalls His Day of Reckoning. Doctor Put Conscience on Hold until War Atrocity Confession Time Came." *The Japan Times Online*.

[71]   D Guyatt. "Deep Black Lies. Unit 731."

during the war ended up in leading positions in medicine and pharmaceutical industry (e.g. The Green Cross Company headed by Naito Ryoichi), and dominated medical science in Japan for the rest of their lives. Most of the victims were communist partisans, ordinary criminals, political dissidents, mentally disabled peasants, and eventually, when these groups run out, local population of the poor and homeless.[72]

In late spring and early summer of the year 1945, Japanese troops began withdrawing from southern China. There were approximately 30,000 American advisers in China with the U.S. Forces China Theater and Chinese Combat Command, including Nisei linguists. Lt. Gen. Albert Wedemeyer and Chiang Kai-shek agreed that after the surrender of Japan, U.S. forces would seize Chinese coastal cities in the event of sudden collapse of Japan. After the surrender of Japan, 3 million Japanese soldiers remained in China and Manchuria, and surrendered to Chiang Kai-shek, as agreed with the U.S. Joint Chief of Staff. The American Dixie Mission was assigned to Yenan in order to find more effective Chinese opposition to the Japanese. Roosevelt Administration wished to see strong China emerging from the war as a counterweight to the USSR and Japan, and backed up Chiang Kai-shek who in their eyes was most likely to succeed.[73] On August 9, 1945, the USSR broke in and invaded Northern China and Manchuria and seized Northern part of Korean peninsula and Sakhalin Island.

Immediately after the surrender of Japan on August 15, 1945, Office for Strategic Service (OSS) Detachment 202 conducted rescue missions for Allied prisoners of war in eight POW camps in China, Korea, Hainan Island, and Formosa. One of the OSS teams accompanied by Nisei linguists went to Manchuria in search

---

[72]   SH Harris. 1999. "Japanese Medical Atrocities in World War II: Unit 731 Was Not an Isolated Aberration." In Tokyo, Japan.

[73]   U.S. Department of State: Office of the Historian. Foreign Relations of the United States, 1969–1976, Volume E-13, Documents on China, 1969–1972, Document 86. Paper Prepared by the National Security Council Staff, Washington, undated.

of senior Allied prisoners held by the Japanese, including Maj. Gen. Jonathan M. Wainwright and British General Arthur E. Percival.[74] Over a thousand prisoners were liberated from the camp, including Maj. Gen. George M. Parker, who recommended the OSS team for Distinguished Service Cross[75].

At the war end, there was substantial problem with evidence regarding Japanese war crimes in occupied territories. On August 15, the Japanese government announced the decision to surrender to the Allied forces and accept the Potsdam Declaration. The decision to destroy all secret documents came a day later. It has to be remembered that in Europe the presence of the U.S. military was much stronger than in the Pacific and therefore securing of the evidence was much more realistic despite Nazi efforts to burn the documents. The first Allied force did not arrive in Japan until August 28. Moreover, the concerned Unit 731 was located in Manchuria, which was by then occupied by the Soviets who seized some of the research on biological and chemical warfare. Despite systematic destruction of Japanese records by the Kwantung Army in the end of the WW2, the Marines and OSS managed to seize large numbers of documents. The main focus of the U.S. authorities was on individuals responsible for Pearl Harbor, mistreatment of U.S. POWs, and war crimes against Caucasian women, especial their exploitation as so-called comfort women for the Japanese Army. In 2000, U.S. Congress finally passed the Japanese Imperial Government Disclosure Act, and the Interagency Working Group was created.

There was no "Doctor trial" with the Japanese doctors who conducted field tests on prisoners of war in China. They got away with it. When confronted by advocacy and human rights groups, the Japanese government insisted these issues had been settled by stipulations of the peace treaty signed in San Francisco in September 1951. The reasons for this stubborn denial of history

---

[74]   James McNaughton. 2006. *Nisei Linguists: Japanese Americans in the Military Intelligence Service during World War II; p 399*. Department of the Army, Washington D.C.

[75]   Ibid; p 400.

in Japan were mainly driven by then conservative ruling party. The general consensus was that the role of Emperor Hirohito in the WW2 is a taboo subject in Japan.[76]

The situation had changed in the 1990's when Japanese scholars and researchers started discussing the topic in the media and the taboo subject was re-opened due to relation to Japanese war crimes in China. The most notorious suspected WW2 criminals who were never punished for their actions were Ishii Shiro of Unit 731, Hatoyama Ichirō (Prime Minister 1954–1956), Ikeda Hayato (Prime Minister 1960–1964), and Kishi Nobusuke (Prime Minister 1957). A convicted Class A war criminal, Shigemitsu Mamoru, a senior diplomat and foreign minister during the war years, regained the foreign minister portfolio in 1954. Transfer of both suspected and convicted war criminals back in positions of power after the war was smooth and undisturbed.[77]

Japanese Emperor Hirohito did not stand trial for war crimes committed by Imperial Japanese Army, but many of the high officials and Army Generals, including Gen. Hideki Tojo, did. When the CIC agents arrived to his house on September 11, 1945, Tojo shot himself before they could arrest him. Tojo recovered to face trial, and eventually was one of those executed for war crimes[78]. Tokyo War Crimes Tribunal resulted in conviction of 25 defendants, whilst the Soviet led Khabarovsk trial brought to trial 5.379 of them and convicted 4.300. The Khabarovsk trial was dismissed by most

---

[76]   E Drea, G Bradsher, R Hanyok, J Lide, M Petersen, and D Yang. 2006. "Nazi War Crimes and Japanese Imperial Government Records Interagency Working Group." In *Researching Japanese War Crimes Records Introductory Essays.* Introduction p. 5. Japanese War Crimes Records at the National Archives: Research Starting Points. Washington D.C.

[77]   Drea E, Bradsher G, Hanyok R, Lide J, Petersen M, Yang D: Researching Japanese War Crimes Records Introductory Essays. Nazi War Crimes and Japanese Imperial Government Records Interagency Working Group. Washington D.C. 2006; Introduction, p 6.

[78]   McNaughton, James C: Nisei Linguists: Japanese Americans in the Military Intelligence service during World War II. Department of the Army, Washington D.C. 2006; p 438.

people in the West as yet another Soviet style kangaroo court and its results were never examined in detail by Western historians.

As per the Institute for Defense Studies and Analyses, Japan does not currently possess any Weapons of Mass Destruction including Biological and Chemical Warfare. This claim disregards Japanese testing of biological and chemical warfare on Allied POWs during the World War Two. The Japanese Biological and Chemical Warfare research was mainly conducted by the Kwantung Army in Northeast China. Medical officer Colonel Shiro Ishii, who was in charge of the Unit 731 in Harbin, Manchuria, since 1935, was the main mastermind of the Japanese Biological Warfare research. Unit 100, commanded by Jiro Wakamatsu, focused on different type of biological warfare – extermination of animals and crops by disease and inducing famine by artificial creation of shortage of food. The main diseases used were cholera, typhoid, anthrax, and bubonic plague; and the main vector used to spread the disease were fleas. Japan only signed the Biological Weapons Convention in 1982 and the Chemical Weapons Convention in 1997, after the sarin attacks in Tokyo.[79]

After the WW2, the only power which wished to pursue a trial against Japanese war criminals in manner similar to the Nuremberg trials with the Nazis was the USA. The Tokyo War Crimes Tribunal began in May 1946 and ended in November 1948. Of 25 defendants, 7 were sentenced to death by hanging and executed, 16 were sentenced to life imprisonment, and 2 received lesser terms. Of those sentenced to life only 4 died in prison. All others were granted clemency.[80]

---

[79]   Shamshad A Khan. 2009. "Japan: CBW. Institute for Defense Studies and Analyses." *CBW Magazine.*

[80]   Drea E, Bradsher G, Hanyok R, Lide J, Petersen M, Yang D: Researching Japanese War Crimes Records Introductory Essays. Nazi War Crimes and Japanese Imperial Government Records Interagency Working Group. Washington D.C. 2006; Introduction, p 6.

THOMAS PERCIVAL'S MEDICAL JURISPRUDENCE AND MEDICAL ETHICS

Percival's Medical jurisprudence or Code of Ethics is the first code of this kind in Europe. This professional code fulfills all criteria defined by Davis: It is a code of ethics; it applies to members of a profession; it applies to all members of that profession, and the scope is limited only to members of the profession. On the other hand, universal moral codes, legal codes, industrial codes, and corporate codes of ethics do not qualify as professional codes of ethics.[81] Before Percival wrote his book, medical ethics in Europe had no authoritative formulation. Since the point of codification is to give law, a code without an authoritative formulation would seem to be no code at all. The fact that there was no formally adopted written code of professional ethics later became the most important argument in the defense of the medical community in Nazi Germany in face of the Nuremberg war crimes tribunal. Any code, including any code of professional ethics, must have a set form.[82] Gentlemen agreements were no longer considered sufficient. English physician Thomas Percival is responsible for two major works on medical ethics: Medical Jurisprudence (1794) and Medical Ethics (1803).

The first of his two works, Medical Jurisprudence, was published in response to a dispute among doctors in a hospital in Manchester after the facility had been swamped by patients with typhus and typhoid. Although the work was not originally intended for wider use but for the hospital staff only, it was brought to the attention of important medical personages and widely discussed within the medical community. A decade later, Percival published his most important work Medical Ethics in which he presents guidelines

---

[81]   M Davis. 2003. "What Can We Learn by Looking for the First Code of Professional Ethics?" *Theoretical Medicine and Bioethics* 24 (5): 433–54.

[82]   Joel Price. 2014. "Writing a Code of Ethics Writing a Code of Ethics." *Scholars Portfolio Education Specialist.*

for conduct in hospital practice, private and general practice, and dealing with apothecaries and legal matters. The Code was also adopted by the American Medical Association in 1847.[83]

Despite major revisions in this code made by AMA in 1903, 1912, 1947, and 1994, the core of the original Percival's work remains the same. The ethical code focuses mainly on conduct of medical professionals to each other and pays little attention to a patient who is mainly seen as a valued paying client who is not supposed to interfere with physician's work. Care for poor patients was the responsibility of the whole faculty and community; and amount of time and resources dedicated to them was subject to many disputes. Increased numbers of doctors allocated to a municipal hospital in Manchester during a typhus epidemic provoked many complaints among attending physicians; and the clash was eventually resolved through implementation of a code.

Medical jurisprudence or the Code of Ethics and Institutes

Percival's Code of Ethics was adopted by the professions of physicians and surgeons; and it teaches that the rules established for hospitals shall be respected in private and general practice as well. It was clearly written with an example of Justinian Code in mind, as stated in the Preface: 'According to the definition of Justinian, however, Jurisprudence may be understood to include moral injunctions as well as positive ordinances.'[84] Every case should be treated with attention, steadiness, and humanity; and confidentiality should always be observed even in the most peculiar circumstances. Vigorous understanding is required at all times and especially in emergencies. For this reason, Percival discourages doctors from drinking even when off duty. Exaggerating of gravity of the patient's condition for the sole purpose of keeping him in doctor's practice or pushing medically unnecessary procedures

---

[83] "Thomas Percival (1740 – 1804)." 2014. *Reynolds Historical Library.*

[84] M Davis. 2003. "What Can We Learn by Looking for the First Code of Professional Ethics?" *Theoretical Medicine and Bioethics* 24 (5): 433–54.

on him is unethical, just like not referring the patient to a more specialized practitioner in cases when the patient's condition requires specialized care. The physician shall never forget to provide faith and comfort to the sick. Any officious interference should be carefully avoided in a case under the charge of another and no selfish conduct pursued, that may directly or indirectly diminish the trust reposed in the physician or surgeon employed.

When a physician or surgeon is called to visit a patient who has been before under the care of another gentleman of the faculty, a consultation with him should be requested if practicable. In larger towns, the distinction between physic (internal medicine) and surgery should be steadily maintained. Consultations should be promoted in difficult or protracted cases as they give rife, energy, and more enlarged views in practice. Should presence of another physician or surgeon be objectionable by the patient, the consultation shall be limited to two or three visits. Theoretical discussions of alternative hypotheses should be avoided in consultations. Seniority of a physician may be determined by the period of his public and acknowledged medical practice in the place where he resides. A regular academic education furnishes the only presumptive evidence of professional ability, although those who do acquire their expertise through experience and practice should not be excluded from fellowship. Visits to the sick should not be unreasonably repeated.

Sir William Temple has asserted that a physician is excused for leaving his patient, when he finds the disease growing desperate, and cannot offer any help to the patient except for charging him his fees. Percival disagrees with Temple on this, and believes continuing visits to terminal patients can be highly useful by obviating despair, alleviating pain, and soothing mental anguish.

A physician or surgeon who officiates for another who is sick or absent should receive the fees accruing from such additional practice. Some general rules should be adopted by the faculty in every town with regards to fees paid by the patients; and these rules shall be adhered to by the faculty members as a matter of honor. All the members of the profession, including apothecaries, as well as physicians and surgeons, together with their wives and children, should be attended gratuitously by any one or more faculty member whose assistance may be required. The use of quack medicines should be discouraged by the whole faculty as injurious to health and disgraceful to the profession; and the effects of well-known active preparations shall not be presented to the patient as quack medicines. No physician or surgeon should dispense a secret nostrum, should it be his invention or exclusive property. If mystery alone gives it value and importance, such craft implies either disgraceful ignorance or fraudulent avarice. When controversies and contentions occur, which cannot be immediately terminated, they should be referred to arbitration of a sufficient number of physicians or of surgeons, according to nature of the dispute. But neither the subject matter nor the adjudication should be communicated to the public, as they may be personally injurious to the individuals concerned, and can hardly fail to hurt the general credit of the faculty.[85]

Percival's Medical Ethics is at least as much about law and custom governing medical practice in England as about what we would now call medical ethics. There was authoritative formulation of Code of medical ethics before Percival's Medical Ethics book. Codification is a way how to give law or any similar system of guidance an authoritative formulation. Even though Percival's Medical Ethics does not fulfill the definition of such code, it certainly was an important step toward developing one. English philosopher Jeremy Benham (1748-1832) attempted to bring standardization of this kind to British law and codification of unwritten rules became main focus of his work.[86]

---

[85]   Thomas Percival. 2014. *Medical Jurisprudence; Or, A Code of Ethics and Institutes Adapted to the Professions of Physic and Surgery (1794).*

[86]   M Davis. 2003. "What Can We Learn by Looking for the First Code of Professional Ethics?" *Theoretical Medicine and Bioethics* 24 (5): 433–54.

OATH OF THE MEDICAL SOCIETY OF NEW YORK

In 1807, the Medical Society of the State of New York introduced a new rule which required all new physicians to sign an oath upon admission to this society. The N.Y. oath required practitioners to practice 'honestly, virtuously, and chastely' and to act with 'fidelity and honor':[87]

> *I do solemnly declare, that I will honestly, virtuously, and chastely conduct myself in the practice of physic and surgery, with the privileges of exercising which profession I am now to be invested; and that I will, with fidelity and honor, do everything in my power for the benefit of the sick committed to my charge.*

---

[87] Daniel Fu-Chang Tsai, and Ding-Shinn Chen. 2003. "An Oath for Bioscientists." *Journal of Biomedical Science* 10: 569–76.

ETHICAL CODE OF THE AMERICAN MEDICAL ASSOCIATION

American Medical Association was the first national professional society in the world to adopt a code of medical ethics. The Code elaborated obligations of physicians to their patients and vice versa, duties of physicians to each other and to the profession at large, duties of physicians in regard to vicarious offices, in consultations, in cases of interference with one another, in regard to pecuniary acknowledgments, and when differences occur between them. The last part details duties of the profession to the public and of obligations of the public to the physicians. The first part stresses the need for secrecy and delicacy when required by peculiar circumstances. Physicians are advised to delegate delivery of unwelcome news to any other person of sufficient judgment and delicacy. Patients who deem incurable shall not be abandoned by their physician who is still obliged to provide hope and alleviate pain and suffering.

In the AMA professional code, patients also have obligations to physicians. First of all, it is the responsibility of patients to choose a physician who has received a regular professional education and whose habits of life are regular and compatible with his professional obligations; and to avoid self-constituted doctors offering infallible remedies. Patients should be open about their symptoms, no matter how embarrassed they may feel about them, because of serious worsening of a disease which might have been readily prevented had timely intimation been given to the physician. Patients should never weary their physician with tedious details of their complaints and unrelated family concerns. The patients should obey the physician's prescriptions not only when it comes to medication, but also with regards to diet, drink, and exercise; and should never send for a consulting physician without the express consent of his own medical attendant. A patient should, after his recovery, entertain a just and enduring sense of the value of the services rendered him by his physician; but when he has to dismiss his physician, justice and common courtesy require that he should declare his reasons for so doing.

In addition to all this, physicians have obligations to each other and to the society as whole. On entering the profession they become entitled to all its privileges and immunities, and should therefore:

> 'observe strictly such laws as are instituted for the government of its members; should avoid all contumelious and sarcastic remarks relative to the faculty, as a body; and while, by unwearied diligence, he resorts to every honorable means of enriching the science, he should entertain a due respect for his seniors, who have, by their labors, brought it to the elevated condition in which he finds it.'

Physicians should

> 'never resort to public advertisements inviting the attention of individuals affected with particular diseases, publicly offering advice and medicine to the poor gratis, or promising radical cures. They also shall not publish cases and operations in the daily prints or suffer such publications to be made, and engage in ordinary practices of empiric.'

Practitioners of medicine and their dependents created a tight-knit community interdependent on each other's services and approval. Physicians and their family members were entitled to services of a practitioner residing near them. They also depended on each other when requesting consultations from colleagues. During consultations, the consulting physician had to behave in a way which would not undermine authority of the attending physician, and they were not supposed to consult any disagreements in front of the patient. Most of this section is dedicated to rules for interaction between neighboring physicians' patients to make sure they do not interfere with each other's affairs. There were also strict rules for any treatment provided free of charge to patients because this behavior was considered fraudulent and harmful to other physicians. Controversies and contentions which cannot be immediately terminated should be referred to court-medical.

> 'A wealthy physician should not give advice gratis to the affluent; because his doing so is an injury to his professional brethren. The office of a physician can never be supported as an exclusively

beneficent one; and it is defrauding, in some degree, the common funds for its support, when fees are dispensed with, which might justly be claimed.'

The duties of physicians to the public mainly include counseling the public and assistance to the authorities on subjects of medical police, public hygiene, and legal medicine. Doctors are also expected to carry out their duties even in situation when their own lives are in jeopardy as a result of public emergency or during an epidemic. The public should award physicians proper honorarium for their work in public interest. In 1847, the American Medical Association was greatly concerned about quack and secret medicines and empirical treatment provided by practitioners without medical education.[88]

Medicine during the Civil War

In 1860, the Union Army only had 30 surgeons and 83 assistants. The Medical Department's expenses for contracted surgeons were relatively high. Civilian doctors were paid $50 if they had to care for 100 or more men; $40 for 50 to 100 men; or $30 if the number of men they cared for was below 50. Some of the young doctors who were still awaiting their examinations and studied contemporary medicine were relatively good and followed closely latest developments in medicine to the benefit of Civil War soldiers. Many major surgeries during the American Civil War were still performed with no anesthesia at all, under the adrenaline rush, mainly due to disruption of supplies. At that time, main anesthetics usable in the field were chloroform and ether. Ether was much less popular because of practicality of logistics and use. Chloroform was simply poured on a cloth and this was placed on the patient's face. Blockade of medical supplies was a major problem especially in the South.

The Geneva Conventions which emerged in Europe as a reaction to the Napoleonic Wars, and demanded neutrality for medical

---

[88]   American Medical Association. 1847. "Code of Medical Ethics of the American Medical Association". American Medical Association Press.

personnel and safe passage of medical supplies were not yet accepted in America by either side. Some older practitioners also refused to use anesthesia during operations because of widespread prejudice. This was mainly the case in obstetrics but also in wartime surgery. No matter the risks and prejudices, two major analgesics spread through America during the Civil War and that was raw opium and morphine, substance isolated from raw opium. Both opium and morphine were mostly administered orally as a powder, applied directly in the wound, or inhaled as smoke. Subcutaneous injections of morphine only came after the Civil War, too late to be of any use for analgesia during surgery. Oral morphine was used for post-operative pain and also for diarrhea, as well as many other ailments including long-term pain management and cough. This practice produced very high numbers of morphine-addicts after the Civil War, especially among women in rural South. Post-operation death rates resulting from infection and hospital gangrene were outrageously high. Even more important problem was lack of aseptic surgical technique.

The era of aseptic surgery only came with Louis Pasteur's discovery of microorganisms and antiseptic methods developed by Joseph Lister, too late for Civil War soldiers.[89] [90] This level of ignorance is rather surprising because the need for clean environment during surgery was well known to many ancient barber-surgeons and medical practitioners who even though had no way of knowing about the link between bacteria and gangrene still understood the importance of washing their hands and using surgical equipment cleaned in 'running water'. Farmers were also familiar with the need for clean surgery. Every animal breeder had experience with neutering farm animals and their reproduction, and it is rather surprising that this knowledge was not applied in military medicine. Using contemporary standards, the AMA medical code of

---

[89]   Mary C Gillett. 2014. "Lawson's Last Years, 1846-1861." In *The Army Medical Department 1818-1865*, edited by David F. Trask. Office of Medical History - U.S. Army Medical Department.

[90]   Mary C Gillett. 2014. "The Civil War, 1861: Many Problems, Few Solutions." In *The Army Medical Department 1818-1865*, edited by David F. Trask. Office of Medical History - U.S. Army Medical Department.

ethics disproportionately protected physicians and their business interests compared to the rights of patients. Probably the most famous victim of 19th century medical malpractice was President James A Garfield who died in 1880 of sepsis 80 days after being shot in his back.[91] None of the two bullets penetrated his vital organs and the patient would have probably been fine if his wound was left to heal conservatively. Unfortunately his physicians took lot of effort to understand pathway of the bullet and at least a dozen of them probed his wound, often with unsterilized fingers and instruments. Unhygienic conditions and heavy food and alcohol ordered by Dr. Willard Bliss did not help to alleviate Garfield's symptoms either. Repeated probing of the wound caused infections which eventually killed the President. At that time, Joseph Lister had been demonstrating his theories on prevention of infection by sterilization of instruments. His discoveries were not that new to the medical community. But in Garfield's case these new techniques were largely ignored. In addition to that, Dr. Bliss fed Garfield large doses of quinine to prevent malaria which was discovered in some puddle nearby and caused a local outbreak. Quinine only caused Garfield even more intestinal cramping.[92] President Garfield's medical bill for all this care amounted to $18.500.

Work of the American Medical Association did not stop with publishing the code of ethics. Soon after, AMA established a board for analysis of quack medicines and nostrums and started educating the public about the dangers of such remedies. In 1858, AMA established Committee on Ethics which soon begun advocating recognition of regularly educated and qualified female physicians. AMA Judicial Council was found in 1873 to deal with ethical and constitutional controversies. Minor changes to the code were made in 1903, and the title was changed to The Principles of Medical Ethics. In 1913, AMA established a specialized department in order to disseminate information about health fraud and quackery. In 1922 amendment made by the Judicial Council outlawed

---

[91]   Amanda Schaffer. 2006. "A President Felled by an Assassin and 1880's Medical Care." *The New York Times*, July 25.

[92]   K Baker. 2011. "The Doctors Who Killed a President." *The New York Times*.

solicitation of patients by physicians. During the Great Depression, it became unethical for any physician to dispose of his or her services to any lay body, organization, group, or individual under the conditions that would permit any of them to receive a profit on the doctor's services; and advocated county medical societies to help share costs for the care of poor patients.[93]

After 1980, clear distinction was made between an ethical code which is not legally binding, and the law. The Association advised physicians not only to oblige by the law but also to report cases of fellow physicians who engage in fraud and deception and other dishonorable behavior. Profession adopted a more proactive approach toward physicians who violated ethical standards and became less worried about the damaged reputation resulting from scandals compared to loss of trust in the profession as whole.

> *Preamble: The medical profession has long subscribed to a body of ethical statements developed primarily for the benefit of the patient. As a member of this profession, a physician must recognize responsibility not only to patients, but also to society, to other health professionals, and to self. The following Principles adopted by the [AMA] are not laws, but standards of conduct which define the essentials of honorable behavior for the physician.*
>
> *II. A physician shall deal honestly with patients and colleagues, and strive to expose those physicians deficient in character or competence, or who engage in fraud or deception.*
>
> *III. A physician shall respect the law and also recognize a responsibility to seek changes in those requirements which are contrary to the best interests of the patient.*
>
> *IV. A physician shall respect the rights of patients, of colleagues, and of other health professionals, and shall safeguard patient confidences within the constraints of the law.*
>
> *V. A physician shall continue to study, apply and advance*

---

[93]   American Medical Association. "Ethics Timeline: 1847 to 1940."

scientific knowledge, make relevant information available to patients, colleagues, and the public, obtain consultation, and use the talents of other health professionals when indicated.

VI. A physician shall, in the provision of appropriate patient care, except in emergencies, be free to choose whom to serve, with whom to associate, and the environment in which to provide medical services.

VII. A physician shall recognize a responsibility to participate in activities contributing to an improved community.

PRUSSIA: ALBERT MOLL'S MEDICAL ETHICS

Prussia is mainly remembered for its achievements on European battlefields, especially due to accomplished military strategist Carl Philipp Gottfried von Clausewitz who stressed the moral and political aspects of war. Prussia's contribution to medical science is unjustly forgotten. In 1891 the Prussian Minister of Interior issued a directive which barred prison physicians from administering tuberculin for the treatment of tuberculosis to prisoners against their will.

In 1898 Albert Neisser, discoverer of Neisseria gonorrheae, conducted an experiment with serum from syphilitic patients. Most of these patients were prostitutes who were unaware of this experiment. None of these patients contracted syphilis from the injections they received without consent but some women later became infected as a result of their career. The trial received lot of attention in the popular media and Neisser had to defend himself in court. Most physicians backed him up in his efforts but there was one who openly objected to the use of patients as experimental subjects for non-therapeutic research without their consent – psychiatrist Albert Moll.[94]

Neisser was fined by the Royal Disciplinary Court, not for questionable science but for failure to obtain informed consent from his patients for this research. The Neisser case triggered discussion within Prussian parliament and the first detailed regulations about non-therapeutic research in Western medicine came from the Prussian minister for religious, educational, and medical affairs in 1900. Emil von Behring argued that self-experimentation should always precede experimentation on patients, and that purely scientific experimentation on human subjects was unethical even with voluntary consent of the subjects. Lawyers believed that non-consensual research fulfilled the criteria

---

[94]   J Vollmann, and R Winau. 1996. "Informed Consent in Human Experimentation before the Nuremberg Code." *British Medical Journal* 313 (7070): 1445-49.

for causing physical injury in criminal law and that scientific value of such experimentation did not serve as mitigation. Informed consent was mandatory and the role of unequal relationship between the physician and his patient was analyzed in thorough detail. The overall conclusion of the Neisser case was that respect for individual rights and morality have the same importance for the good of mankind as medical and scientific progress. In 1900 the Minister for religious, educational and medical affairs issued a directive which demanded informed consent of the patient for all medical interventions other than diagnostic, treatment, and immunization and documentation of all such experiments. The directive was not legally binding and its enforceability remained questionable. [95]

Barbara Elkeles in her study on practices in human experimentation in Imperial Germany pointed out, that medical researchers were more concerned about science than safety of their subjects. This attitude stemmed from authoritarian culture of German universities and hospitals. Doctors in Imperial Germany greatly benefited from compulsory health insurance for workers which brought in their offices many people from lower income classes who otherwise would hardly consulted a doctor. This insurance scheme tied German physicians to the state more than to their patients because they were paid through insurance funds and some were directly employed by them. This economic setup made conditions of German physicians very different from those of their British and American colleagues. Whilst in 1885 the percentage of German population insured by state was about 9%, in the beginning of the First World War this number increased to about one third of the total population including family members and dependents.

---

[95] J Vollmann, and R Winau. 1996. "Informed Consent in Human Experimentation before the Nuremberg Code." *British Medical Journal* 313 (7070): 1445–49.

In 1902 Albert Moll (1862 – 1939)[96] a psychiatrist from Berlin published 650 pages long handbook 'Physician's ethics' in which he summarized history of professional duties and medical ethics in Germany from the foundation of the Second Reich in 1871 to the First World War. Moll was well recognized for his works in sexuology, sexual forensics, and hypnosis, and got involved in many fierce academic debates with his contemporaries. Unlike most, Moll rejected then very popular teachings of Sigmund Freud and had no respect for him as a person, either. Some authors, such as Paul Weindling, traced the inclination of German medicine to Social Darwinism and eugenics to the wars for German unification and efforts of medical profession to gain more social power.

Professional secrecy was becoming a serious problem in Imperial Germany because protection of individual patients was in conflict with some public interests. The state eventually got its way to protect the society from spread of venereal and other contagious diseases. Introduction of anesthesia in late 1840's and antiseptic techniques in surgery in late 1860's led to rapid development of surgical techniques. This consequently stirred discussions whether it is permissible to perform surgery on a patient who did not give consent to it. The physicians mostly could not see any problem in doing so, as long as the insurance fund did not object, whilst lawyers were in their opinions more split due to concerns about injury to the patient. The first significant victory of the state against the people who did not consent to a medical procedure was compulsory vaccination against smallpox in 1874.

Professional ethics in Imperial Germany was entangled in many social and legal issues, from 'truth-telling' on deathbed to treatment of women who underwent illegal abortions, and palliative care for the dying. Moll based his work on contractual relationship between the doctor and his client which was in direct conflict with paternalistic medicine funded by insurance funds; and engaged in debates on hot topics of those days such as

---

[96] Durham University. 2014. "Moll Project. Sexuology, Medical Ethics, and Occultism."

experimentation on hospital patients, and the 'trade' of foreign private patients between agents and medical consultants. Moll collected evidence of unethical practices of his colleagues and became one of the most outspoken critics of eugenic sterilization after the introduction of the Nuremberg Laws. He did not win many friends for himself in the medical community, but the lawyers accepted his works with great seriousness and appreciation. Moll was especially concerned about many bacteriological experiments within hospitals including infection of dying patients with gonorrhea. Instead of writing a philosophical manuscript, he appealed to intuitive common sense which doctors shared with laymen, and rejected popular standpoints of that time that experiments on dying patients are acceptable because they help future patients, and that refusal of treatment to people with hereditary disabilities is beneficial to society because it prevents the disease to be passed down. Moll believed that the role of physician was that of a healer, and that experiments which would harm an individual patient would negate this commitment.

Moll presented his work in more legal then philosophical sense, and thought about the doctor-patient relationship more like a contract with duties and rights for both sides. Some thought the project was overambitious in its comprehensiveness, and especially in content which went often against the tide and against the deep currents in German society. In his works, Moll focused on doctor-client relationship, as he called the patient, and also discussed other forms of medical practice, such as risky surgical interventions as well as other morally dangerous practices; the role of health insurance system; the role of physicians in the state sector, court service, and insurance organizations; and research on animal and human subjects. Finally, he mentioned the need to teach medical ethics as inherent part of curriculum at medical schools. Moll rejected Kant's and Fichte's opinion that truthfulness is an unconditional duty in any situation as unsuitable for medical practice. The exceptions he saw were always in the best interest of the patient, e.g. when there was a risk of suicide if the patient had been told prognosis too dire to bear. Restrictions on truthfulness were also made toward the terminally ill, as 'cancer patient gains nothing from knowing his malady'.

In 1895, Adolf Jost in his paper 'The right to death' called for decriminalization of euthanasia which in some cases is desirable for both the incurable ill patient and the society. The law could later be extended to euthanasia of incurably mentally ill patients without their consent. Moll firmly rejected such ideas as inadmissible from the point of view of criminal law as well as general morality and used the argument which is now known as the 'slippery slope'. Moll advocated generous use of painkillers in terminal patients even when this practice eventually led to unconsciousness. His understanding was that this practice is part of palliative care. In Moll's opinion, 'heroic' treatment efforts were not consistent with medical ethics as according to Moll the contract was with the patient and not with his relatives. Experimental treatment on dying patients was entirely unacceptable and shameful act of brutality.

Moll also discussed in detail procedure perforation of fetus or craniotomy in situations when the fetus could not be delivered. He argued that mother's life has a priority because an infant is not an independent human being and Cesarean section at that time still carried a risk about ten percent mortality for the mother. From ethical and legal perspective, this procedure was permitted as emergency self-defense. Fetotomy is also practiced in veterinary medicine in situations when normal delivery is not possible because of malformed or overgrown fetus, due to pathologies of pelvis of the mother, and when Cesarean section cannot be performed. Other physicians at that time would perform Cesarean section even against the mother's will or make decision on her behalf without asking. In this sense, Moll's respect for patient's autonomy was for his time extraordinary.

In late 19th century Prussia, about three to five hundred thousand abortions were performed every year even though it was illegal to do so. Women were rarely prosecuted for undergoing abortion. The number of criminal convictions was about one thousand a year. Moll was rather sympathetic to women who opted for early abortion because they were raped or because they had too many children to support. In his opinion, the physician had no duty to disclose such information about his patient to the police. Moll's book contained collection of about 600 research papers on therapeutic and non-therapeutic research from Europe, Russia, United States, Chile, and Egypt, and documented how patients were being harmed or at least molested or exposed to risks through experimentation, often without their knowledge. Most of this research was performed on institutionalized persons in orphanages and prisons and Moll did not conceal his outrage about such practice. List of unethical practices of fellow doctors did not help him to gain popularity even though he was careful enough to omit names. The authorities then attempted to use Moll's research for the book as grounds for prosecution of doctors who were engaging in unethical practices, but Moll was very reluctant to provide this material as he mainly sought amendment of regulations on human experimentation rather than persecution of fellow physicians. After this, Moll mainly focused on sexual forensics and hypnosis, largely ignored by the medical community. His work on medical ethics made headlines once more due to a series of libel suits with colleagues. The trials were widely reported but did not help Moll's reputation at all. Moll's detailed account what medical ethics should look like was marginalized and forgotten. Others got their way.[97]

---

[97]   AH Maehle. 2012. "God's Ethicist: Albert Moll and His Medical Ethics in Theory and Practice." In *Medical History*, 56 (2):217–36. Published by Cambridge University Press.

IMPERIAL HEALTH COUNCIL ON MEDICAL EXPERIMENTATION

The Nuremberg Code from 1947 is generally believed to be the first ethical code on human experimentation. During the Nuremberg trial, doctors who were engaging in horrible atrocities during the war were trying to excuse themselves from responsibility by claims that there were no rules for human experimentation at that time in Germany, and that they only did the same thing which was happening elsewhere. Whilst it is true that eugenic laws were indeed in force in many states in the USA, it has to be stressed that regulations regarding medical experimentation did indeed exist in Germany since late 19th century.

In 1926 Much, author who focused his work on Hippocrates, suggested the use of prisoners and asylum inmates for experimental infections[98], but did not get very far with his request. Reason for this was very likely in the strict safety mindset and system of social and health insurance implemented in Bismarck's Germany 1838-1884. The accident rate in dangerous industries such as construction, railroads, and coal mining, was very low, much lower than in the USA at that time. Costs relating to liabilities for injuries were much lower because less people felt the urge to pursue their claims through litigation.[99] In 1930 the Imperial Health Council (Reichsgesundheitsrat) issued new guidelines for experiments on humans. In a letter to prison service officials in July 1931, the Prussian minister of justice stressed that according to these guidelines experiments on prisoners were not permissible, not even with the inmates' consent.

---

[98]   C Timmermann. 2001. "A Model for the New Physician: Hippocrates in Interwar Germany." In *Reinventing Hippocrates*, 302–24. Centre for the History of Science, Technology and Medicine, University of Manchester.

[99]   JM Kleeberg. 2003. "From Strict Liability to Workers' Compensation: The Prussian Railroad Law, the German Liability Act, and the Introduction of Bismarck's Accident Insurance in Germany, 1838-1884." *International Law and Politics* 36: 53–132.

Circular of the Reich minister of the interior: guidelines for new therapy and human experimentation, 1931:

Prussian medicine was heavily paternalistic and closely tied to interests of the state. As pointed out by Albert Moll, people in institutions were often utilized for clinical experiments without their consent. In the context of political reform of criminal law in Germany, the Reich government issued detailed guidelines for therapeutic research and human experimentation. The guidelines distinguished between therapeutic and non-therapeutic research, and emphasized the importance of informed consent of the patient with the experiment.

The regulations were based on beneficence, non-maleficence, and patients' autonomy. New experimental treatment can only be administered without the patient's consent or proxy consent which has been given in a clear and undebatable manner following appropriate information only if it is urgently required to save the patient's life or prevent severe damage to his health. Non-therapeutic research is under no circumstances permissible without consent. Written documentation and clear structure of responsibility is always required for each trial. The structure of the norm as well as hierarchical model was adopted from the directive originally enacted in 1900. Just as it was formulated in the Nuremberg Code after the Second World War, the 1931 guideline required cost-benefit calculation, detailed research plan, and completed tests on animals in order to minimize risks for human research subjects. Experimentation on dying patients was absolutely prohibited and any exploitation of social or economic needs was rejected in testing new therapies. [100]

In the context of these detailed existing regulations it is hard to understand how it is possible that these new rules were reverted so suddenly and so quickly, with no resistance from the medical community whatsoever. Moll's book on medical ethics which widely advocated patient's autonomy was by the 1930's almost

---

[100]   J Vollmann, and R Winau. 1996. "Informed Consent in Human Experimentation before the Nuremberg Code." *British Medical Journal* 313 (7070): 1445–49.

forgotten. Although it was translated and published in 1903 and 1904 in Russia, in Germany the book never saw second edition. End of Weimar Republic and establishment of Hitler's Third Reich swept the 1931 regulations on medical research on human subjects out of public sight for next fifteen years.

HITLER'S GESUNDHEIT

In 1933, German doctors adopted a very different approach to medical ethics which substantially drifted away from the interest of the patient to the interest of the Nazi state and society. The state desired to purify its own population and improve the race to keep the nation healthy and energetic and free from burdensome lower quality human stock. The demand for elimination of 'bad genes' and 'racial pollution' was by no means new. By that time, eugenics was well established science widely accepted in the scientific and medical community. There was nothing controversial about eugenics at all: it was freely discussed in scientific conferences, articles on improvement of race were plentiful in scientific journals, and there was no public outcry against the efforts to suppress reproduction rate of certain unpopular population groups.

Nazi policy on the improvement of national health stemmed from British and American eugenics. There was nothing particularly controversial about it at that time. The founder of eugenics Francis Galton who was the most prolific author on this topic and who published dozens of pamphlets and articles on eugenics through late 19th and early 20th century was not living in hiding. He was the one who was primarily responsible for the slow shift from theoretical science to practical implementation of policy of sterilization of the 'feeble-minded', 'morons', and 'idiots'. Sterilization laws were already implemented in many American states, although they were used relatively scarcely compared to what was just about to come. At least in theory, court order was required to perform sterilization on a patient who did not give consent to it. By that time, the Indiana sterilization laws were enacted (1907), challenged as unconstitutional (1921), and reversed by a decision of Supreme Court in Virginia in the Buck vs. Bell case in 1927.[101]

---

[101]   U.S. Supreme Court. 1927. *Buck v. Bell*. U.S. Supreme Court.

Implementation of eugenic laws legally binding for physicians in Nazi Germany

December 31, 1931	**SS Engagement and Marriage Order**: In order to transform SS into the organizational, ideological, and racial-biological elite of German Volk, Himmler had to recruit pure-blood members and make sure they find themselves racially pure women and advance biological up-breeding of the SS.[102]
March 23, 1933 Amendment to the Weimar Constitution	**'Act for the Removal of the Distress of the People and the Reich'** (the Enabling Act, Ermächtigungsgesetz): the government of the Reich was to be vested with almost unlimited powers to enact laws, even in cases where the legislation encroached on core provisions of the Constitution. This was the next step towards the 'Führer state' and abolition of parliamentary democracy and the rule of law. Although the NSDAP-led government had a stable working majority in the Reichstag, the National Socialists aspired to formalize their absolute de facto political power by means of an amendment to the Weimar Constitution.[103]

---

[102]   "SS Marriage Order (December 31, 1931). Document 2284-PS [The History, Mission, and Organization of the Schutzstaffeln of the NSDAP, Compiled on the Commission of the Reichsführer-SS by the SS-Standartenführer Gunter d'Alquen, 1939], Pp. 976-77." 1931. In United States Chief Counsel for the Prosecution of Axis Criminality, Nazi Conspiracy and Aggression, Volume IV. Washington, DC: United States Government Printing Office, 1946.

[103]   "Law to Remove the Distress of the People and the Reich (Enabling Act)." 2014. reprinted in U.S. Department of State, Division of European Affairs, National Socialism. Basic Principles, their Application by the Nazi Party's Foreign Organizations, and the Use of Germans Abroad for Nazi Aims. Washington, DC: United States Government Printing Office, 1943, Appendix, Document 11, pp. 217-18.

April 7, 1933 The Reich Ministry of the Interior under the leadership of Wilhelm Frick (1877-1946)	**Law for the Restoration of the Professional Civil Service"** (the Civil Service Law): This law excluded all racial and political 'enemies' of the regime from the civil service and required all public sector employees to provide certification of Aryan ancestry [Ariernachweis] documenting their racial purity.[104]
Passed: 14 July 1933 In effect: January 1, 1934 Main propagator: Rudolf Heß (1894-1987) Signed by: Adolf Hitler (Chancellor) Wilhelm Frick (Ministry of Interior) Dr. Gürtner (Ministry of Justice)	**'Law for the Prevention of Offspring with Hereditary Diseases'**: Although the National Socialists rated the Jews as the most dangerous racial 'enemy' of the German Volk, their racial policies also extended to other biologically-defined groups (1. Congenital mental deficiency, 2. Schizophrenia, 3. Manic-depression, 4. Hereditary epilepsy, 5. Hereditary St. Vitus' Dance (Huntington's Chorea), 6. Hereditary blindness, 7. Hereditary deafness, 8. Serious hereditary physical deformity). This law sought to prevent the possible transmission of hereditary diseases through forced sterilization. Individual cases were reviewed by Eugenics Courts consisting of lawyers and doctors loyal to the regime. Although this program was largely suspended in 1939 the Eugenics Courts ordered the "Hitler cut" [Hitlerschnitt] to be carried out on about 400,000 individuals up to the end of the war.[105]
Enacted: 15 Sep 1935 Passed during the Seventh Reich Party Rally of the NSDAP in	The **'Law for the Protection of German Blood and German Honor'** ('Blood Protection Law') aimed to isolate the Jews racially and socially by prohibiting them from marrying or having sexual relations with non-Jews. In addition, Jews were prohibited from employing Aryan housemaids

---

[104] "German History in Documents and Images: Volume 7. Nazi Germany, 1933-1945; Law for the Restoration of the Professional Civil Service (April 7, 1933)."

[105] "Law for the Prevention of Offspring with Hereditary Diseases (July 14, 1933). Document 3067-PS, Pp. 880-83". In US Chief Counsel for the Prosecution of Axis Criminality, Nazi Conspiracy and Aggression. Volume 5, Washington, DC: United States Government Printing Office, 1946.

Nuremberg Adolf Hitler, Wilhelm Frick	younger than 45. They were also barred from flying the new, official swastika flag. The 'Reich Citizenship Law' stripped all Jews of the political rights deriving from German Reich citizenship and relegated them to the status of second-class citizens. In the following months, the regime used this legal demotion to push the Jews out of a number of professions, occupations, and programs of study for which Reich citizenship was required.[106]
Enacted: 18 Oct 1935	**'Law for the Protection of the Hereditary Health of the German People'** **(Marriage Health Law)** banned union between Aryans and non-Aryans and made it a national duty for Aryans to have as many children as possible. Nuremberg racial laws prohibited marriage and sexual relations between Germans and Gypsies, Jews, and Blacks and openly discriminated against non-Germans and the handicapped.
Enacted: 14 Nov 1935 Adolf Hitler, Wilhelm Frick, Rudolf Heß	An official definition of a full Jew or a mixed-breed [Mischling] was provided by the **'First Regulation to the Reich Citizenship Law'** of November 14, 1935 (or the Implementing Decree of November 14, 1935).[107]

---

[106] "The Reich Citizenship Law of September 15, 1935, and the First Regulation to the Reich Citizenship Law of November 14, 1935. Documents 1416-PS and 1417-PS, Pp. 7-10." 2014. In United States Chief Counsel for the Prosecution of Axis Criminality, Nazi Conspiracy and Aggression, Volume IV. Washington, DC: United States Government Printing Office, 1946.

[107] "The Reich Citizenship Law of September 15, 1935, and the First Regulation to the Reich Citizenship Law of November 14, 1935 Documents 1416-PS and 1417-PS, Pp. 7-10." 2014. In United States Chief Counsel for the Prosecution of Axis Criminality, Nazi Conspiracy and Aggression, Volume IV. Washington, DC: United States Government Printing Office, 1946.

Nuremberg Racial Laws thus did not draw the attention they should have because there was nothing particularly abominable about them, at least not in the eyes of those who formed public opinion at that time. The medical oath itself did not change, but the reasoning Nazi doctors were using to justify sterilization and killing some of their patients deserves attention. Widespread acceptance of eugenics and racial theory was not invented by Hitler; he only used it against a specific unpopular ethnic group which was not in fact a primary target of eugenic theories for racial improvement. The primary targets were the 'feeble-minded', 'morons', and 'idiots', people with hereditary diseases, convicted criminals, and former African slaves.

The problem was not the medical oath – that remained intact, but its interpretation was twisted. To some groups of people the Hippocratic Oath no longer applied. Hippocratic principles were completely turned around to conform to the interest of society rather than an individual. Life was divided into that which was worth protection and that which had to be suppressed or eliminated in order to produce better race, and to improve overall health status of the nation and its gene pool. Life unworthy to live was then precisely defined in law and utilized for the benefit of those who still had value. Even though eugenics was long accepted in the scientific community, and it was the Americans who implemented some aspects of it in practice through compulsory sterilization of certain individuals, it was the Nazis who took the extra step, and implemented series of laws which were primarily intended to eliminate certain population subgroups completely.

Hanauska and Abel[108] examined two most popular theories on decline of German medicine in the 1930's – 'slippery slope' and 'sudden subversion'. The first theory, slippery slope, connotes a gradual slide which is not noticed by most at first but becomes deadly when suddenly all footing is lost. Life unworthy to be lived

---

[108]   Hanauske-Abel, HM: Not a Slippery Slope or Sudden Subversion: German Medicine and National Socialism in 1933. A5 Medicine & Global Survival 1996; Vol. 3.

first only included those incurably ill, then those mentally ill who presented too high burden for German social and healthcare system, then political and racial undesirables, and eventually all non-Germans. The second theory, sudden subversion, conveys forced takeover of the profession's leadership and values. This concept is still very popular among German physicians because it shifts guilt from medical professionals to political leadership. Both concepts imply that medical profession was mere victim of circumstances and political system imposed which was by Hitler.

The authors reviewed documents published in German medical journals during 1933 and came to a conclusion that none of these theories applies because it was the German medical community itself which set its own course, and in some respects even outpaced the new government. The relationship between the medical community and government profoundly changed in 1933. In the early 1930's Munchener Medizinische Wochenschrift promoted nationalistic, anti-Semitic, and eugenic ideas so aggressively that in 1935 neighboring Czechoslovakia categorized the journal as fascist and banned its distribution.

Hitler was elected Chancellor on January 1, 1933. On 21 March 1933, the Chancellor and the Reich President open the session of the new parliament in the Potsdam Garrison Church. Dr. A. Stauder, the president of the two largest German medical associations, met with other National Socialists in Munich. After the meeting he telegraphed Hitler immediately that "the principal professional organizations in Germany gladly welcome the firm determination of the Government of National Renewal to build a true community of all ranks, professions, and classes, and they gladly place themselves at the service of this great patriotic task".

Prussian Chamber of Physicians and German Society for Internal Medicine were similarly delighted that democratic government is over and expressed their dedication to Hitler's National Health program. Apart from the fact that German physicians greatly benefited from the fact that Jewish doctors were banned from practicing medicine and the positions they held thus remained vacant, free to be taken over by Aryans, pro-Nazi doctors also could take jobs in newly established institutions such as Dachau and

Sachsenhausen. About 17% of all physicians in Germany in 1933 were Jewish, so the number of vacated positions after they were banned from practicing medicine was very significant. By end of 1933 several dozen concentration camps were in operation and lucrative positions were advertised in well-established medical journals. Physicians who worked in these legal institutions not only took up these jobs voluntarily; they accepted the most active role in the holocaust by direct participation in falsifying medical records and suppressing physical findings of malnutrition and torture.

Active role of medical and scientific community in implementation of racial hygiene is indisputable, as obvious from a petition to the Ministry of Interior of the Weimar Republic sent by the Deutscher Ärztevereinsbund in November 1932. The Ministry reacted promptly and appointed Professor Rudin a chairman of an advisory panel for formulation of eugenic legislation. The purity of German race and the need to dispose of non-German and unhealthy elements was well recognized by Nazi physicians. Those who objected the whole concept of Nazi genetic health and eugenic medicine were few and far between. For most of them, it was financially very convenient to join the crowd. By end of 1935, income of Aryan physicians increased by 25%. Hanauske-Abel argued that even though the change within German medical community was rather abrupt and came in relatively short period of time from late 1932 to mid-1933 it was not imposed from outside but from within. The author emphasized the role of The Kaiser-Wilhelm Society for the Advancement of Sciences and prominent German physicians who were determined to make the sole objective of German medicine to systematically serve the Reich[109].

Robert Jay Lifton suggested that Nazi doctors perverted medical ethics by valuing the health of the Volk over that of the individual. Hippocratic principles of medical ethics are associated with emphasis on the interest of individual patient and the principle of doing no harm. In the 1920's, neo-Hippocratic

---

[109]   Hanauske-Abel, HM: Not a Slippery Slope or Sudden Subversion: German Medicine and National Socialism in 1933. A5 Medicine & Global Survival 1996; Vol. 3.

movement was gaining popularity in Britain, France and Germany. There was nothing substantially different in their training in medical ethics. Whilst in Britain and France the emphasis was on the rights of an individual, in Germany economic hardships resulting from humiliation by the Versailles Treaty, creation of the Weimar Republic through 1918 revolution, and war reparations imposed by the Allies created a mindset of the need to ensure national survival at higher than individual level.

The memory of German unification under Bismarck was still very fresh. The slaughter of the First World War not only caused many people to meet an unnatural death, it also stalled demographic growth because of the sheer number of young people killed and because of economic austerity which followed after the war. This could explain enhanced need for ethnic purification and national revival under existential threat. German mythology played crucial role in wide acceptance of Blood Protection Law and similar measures. The Nuremberg racial laws were consistent with the message passed down through medieval heroic sagas and ancient German mythology and popular fairy-tales.

Timmermann[110] in his paper on Hippocrates in interwar Germany stated that current interpretation of Hippocrates ascribes higher meaning to the Hippocratic Oath because of civil rights movements of the 1960's and does not apply to a professional ideology which is highly interest-driven. The doyen of German interwar Hippocratism, August Bier (1861-1949), a recognized and admired surgeon, became a patron of unorthodox practices such as homeopathy and natural healing. Much, another interwar German author who focused his interest on Hippocrates claimed that in the person of Hippocrates, several ancient high cultures culminated. Not only had he represented the best of ancient Greece, Egyptian and Indian cultures manifested in his works also. Both Much and Bier saw conflict between healing and medical science and between rules of nature and natural laws. This interpretation would give

---

[110]   C Timmermann. 2001. "A Model for the New Physician: Hippocrates in Interwar Germany." In *Reinventing Hippocrates*, 302–24. Centre for the History of Science, Technology and Medicine, University of Manchester.

Hippocratic Oath a completely different meaning than that which is attributed to the oath today. From this point of view it is not surprising that German physicians drifted away from Hippocratic principles of focus on individual patient at all. Both Much and Bier believed that medicine could not simply be learned because the ideal physician would be part philosopher and part priest rather than simply an expert in health management obsessed with biological explanations of life and death. To add economic motivator to ideology, Reich doctors found their autonomy severely restricted by insurance funds. These funds provided access to healthcare to patients who would have otherwise hardly consulted any doctor at all. Psychological factor of a white coat comes in also at this point because people with very limited previous experience with physicians are more likely to be receptive to authority of a medical professional. People who were used to pay physicians directly would hardly agree to pay for being harmed by a service provider. New naive patients reacted differently.

The T4 euthanasia program should have created a moral dilemma for German physicians because of direct conflict with the Hippocratic principle of inflicting no harm to the patient. For most of them it did not pose any trouble at all because non-Germans were no longer patients but only research subjects or genetic waste not worth any investment at all. The reasons for this can be partially learned from the statements of Nazi doctors who were charged with crimes against humanity at the Nuremberg tribunal. Nazi doctors argued that the whole idea of eugenics and compulsory sterilization of defective humans came from the USA, and they only adopted the same principle. This was not exactly the case because in the USA eugenic movement was already on the decline without reaching the stage of mass murder of its own undesired citizens.

Sterilization laws were in force for much longer period of time (since 1907) affecting potentially many more people. America was undergoing profound changes because of liberation of former slaves and their gradual adaptation and slow integration in society which was by no means clash-free. The country also had very serious problem with displaced and homeless people who fell victim to the 1930's depression, series of bad harvests and rapidly progressing industrialization of agriculture, and rampant organized crime in many cities at time when FBI was still in its early years of consolidation. Significant percentage of forcibly sterilized people and especially women were black. But it has to be stressed that despite the popularity of eugenic movement, reluctance of other physicians and scientists to openly condemn eugenics and especially negative eugenics (sterilizations and euthanasia), and the whole madness of racial hygiene and consolidation of totalitarian power in Germany, the total numbers of all non-consensual sterilizations in America did not exceed 15.000 by 1929 and 60.000 people over several decades. In comparison to this, the Germans managed to sterilize about 400.000 people during just a few years in a country which was much smaller and much less ethnically diverse.

Other authors, such as Drobniewski, pointed out psychological factors such as fear of punishment and learned inhibition to commit murder, elitism, legal protection of perpetrators and their conditioning with rewards. An elitist can justify genocide in his own mind due to inherent feelings of self-righteousness, racial advancement, moral superiority, and group loyalty. Dissidents within the medical community were ostracized for dishonoring the German medical profession. These measures, from character assassination to loss of livelihood, served as a very powerful deterrent for all others who would dare to have different opinion than the well-off majority. Hanauske-Abel was barred from practicing medicine for publishing the article on Slippery slope or sudden subversion cited above as late as in 1980.[111]

In 1920, Karl Binding and Alfred Hoche published book 'The permission to destroy life unworthy of life' in which they argued that mercy killing of people who are 'mentally dead' with little or no prospect of improvement is both ethical and legal. The nation did not yet recover from the horrors of the First World War in which their bravest young men died for the Volk whilst the nation was now forced to care for the incurably sick and the

---

[111]   F Drobniewski. 1993. "Why Did Nazi Doctors Break Their 'Hippocratic' Oaths?" *Journal of the Royal Society of Medicine* 86: 541–43.

deranged at times when normal and sane people were starving. Patients who did not recover from chronic shell-shock, now known as post-traumatic stress disorder (PTSD) were filling lunatic asylums and their prospects of recovery were almost nil. It requires lot of cynicism to describe war veterans disabled by war as burden to society. Between 1924 and 1929 the number of psychiatric patients rose dramatically, from 185,397 to more than 300,000 without commensurate increase in bed capacity. It became a generally accepted truth that caring for chronic or geriatric patients represented a 'luxury that Germany could not afford'. A financially constrained nation was in the process of 'caring itself to death.'

Already during the First World War, 140,234 psychiatric asylum patients died, about half of this number as a direct result of hunger, disease and neglect.[112] Paul Weindling suggested that for Binding and Hoche 'the war destroyed the value attached to individual life, shifting the emphasis to collective national survival'. The first volume of a series of books on 'The Doctor's Eternal Mission' (Ewiges Arzttum) contained a collection of Hippocratic texts edited by Ernst Robert von Grawitz, chief physician of the SS, with introduction by Heinrich Himmler. By 1939, Hippocratic Oath completely lost its original meaning.[113]

---

[112]   JR Silver. 2003. "The Decline of German Medicine, 1933-45." *J R Coll Physicians Edinb* 33: 54–66.

[113]   C Timmermann. 2001. "A Model for the New Physician: Hippocrates in Interwar Germany." In *Reinventing Hippocrates*, 302–24. Centre for the History of Science, Technology and Medicine, University of Manchester.

WORLD MEDICAL ASSOCIATION – THE DECLARATION OF GENEVA (1948)

After the Second World War, in reaction to atrocities committed by German physicians on Jews, non-German nationals, political undesirables, homosexuals, women who remained unmarried because of stigmatization by Hitler cut, prisoners of war, especially those from the Eastern front, people from mental health institutions, and other categories of undesirables, a new set of rules on clinical research on humans was put in place.

The Declaration of Geneva[114] was adopted by the 2nd General Assembly of the World Medical Association in September 1948 in Geneva, Switzerland; and amended by the 22nd General Assembly in Sydney in August 1968; then in 1983 in Venice; in 1994 in Stockholm; in May 2005 in France, and the last time by the 173rd WMA Council Session at the same place a year later.

Declaration of Geneva is a Pledge taken by a graduate being admitted as a member of the medical profession and it replaces the Hippocratic Oath. Although widely in use, it is not legally binding. Many universities use a different type of oath upon commencing medical practice. As per this pledge, physicians are not supposed to take into consideration age, disease, disability, creed, political affiliation, ethnic origin, nationality, race, sexual orientation, or social standing; and to use their medical knowledge to violate human rights and civil liberties. This medical oath is too vague to address any practical problems medical profession faced in the past and which it was meant to rectify.

The Declaration of Geneva, just like previous oaths and ethical codes, stressed the importance of professional honor with regards to knowledge and respect to colleagues and teachers, focus on patient and confidentiality of anything what is shared between the physician and the patient.

---

[114] World Medical Association, Geneva. 1948. "The Declaration of Geneva."

I SOLEMNLY PLEDGE to consecrate my life to the service of humanity;

I WILL GIVE to my teachers the respect and gratitude that is their due;

I WILL PRACTISE my profession with conscience and dignity;

THE HEALTH OF MY PATIENT will be my first consideration;

I WILL RESPECT the secrets that are confided in me, even after the patient has died;

I WILL MAINTAIN by all the means in my power, the honor and the noble traditions of the medical profession;

MY COLLEAGUES will be my sisters and brothers;

I WILL NOT PERMIT considerations of age, disease or disability, creed, ethnic origin, gender, nationality, political affiliation, race, sexual orientation, social standing or any other factor to intervene between my duty and my patient;

I WILL MAINTAIN the utmost respect for human life;

I WILL NOT USE my medical knowledge to violate human rights and civil liberties, even under threat;

I MAKE THESE PROMISES solemnly, freely and upon my honor.

INTERNATIONAL CODE OF MEDICAL ETHICS (1949)

The international code of medical ethics was adopted by the 3rd General Assembly of the World Medical Association in London, England, in October 1949, and amended in Sydney, Australia, in August 1968; then in 1983 in Venice, Italy; and eventually in 2006 in Pilanesberg, South Africa. According to this code, a physician shall always exercise his or her independent professional judgment and maintain the highest standards of professional conduct; respect a competent patient's right to accept or refuse treatment; not allow his or her judgment to be influenced by personal profit or unfair discrimination; be dedicated to providing competent medical service in full professional and moral independence, with compassion and respect for human dignity; deal honestly with patients and colleagues; and report to the appropriate authorities those physicians who practice unethically or incompetently or who engage in fraud or deception; not receive any financial benefits or other incentives solely for referring patients or prescribing specific products; respect the rights and preferences of patients, colleagues, and other health professionals; recognize his or her important role in educating the public but should use due caution in divulging discoveries or new techniques or treatment through non-professional channels; certify only that which he or she has personally verified; strive to use health care resources in the best way to benefit patients and their community; seek appropriate care and attention if he or she suffers from mental or physical illness; and respect the local and national codes of ethics.

Physicians' duties to patients include the obligation to always respect human life and to act in the best interest of the patient when providing medical care.

Physicians owe their patients complete loyalty and all the scientific resources available to them. Whenever an examination or treatment is beyond the physician's capacity, he or she should consult with or refer to another physician who has the necessary ability.

A physician shall always respect patient's right to confidentiality. It is ethical to disclose confidential information when the patient consents to it or when there is a real and imminent threat of harm to the patient or to others and this threat can be only removed by a breach of confidentiality.

Physicians shall give emergency care as a humanitarian duty unless they are assured that others are willing and able to give such care. In situations when a physician is acting for a third party, he or she shall ensure that the patient has full knowledge of that situation.

A physician shall not enter into a sexual relationship with his or her current patient or into any other abusive or exploitative relationship.

A physician shall behave towards colleagues as he or she would have them behave towards him or her; and shall not undermine the patient-physician relationship of colleagues in order to attract patients.

When medically necessary, physician shall communicate with colleagues who are involved in the care of the same patient. This communication should respect patient confidentiality and be confined to necessary information.[115]

After the War, all doctors in West Germany had to retake the new WMA Oath. Only a tiny minority of Nazi doctors was punished for crimes against humanity; most were allowed to continue their practices.

---

[115]   World Medical Association. 1949. "International Code of Medical Ethics". World Medical Association.

THE LOUIS LASAGNA OATH

In 1964, Academic Dean of the School of Medicine at Tufts University Louis Cesare Lasagna (1923 – 2003) revised Hippocratic Oath and modified it for modern medicine. The Oath was since adopted by many medical schools where it effectively replaced the World Medical Association from 1948. Dr. Lasagna was an internationally recognized expert in clinical pharmacology who graduated from Rutgers University in 1943 and earned his medical degree from Columbia in 1947 before he moved on to Harvard Medical School where he completed clinical research fellowship in anesthesia. In 1954 he joined John Hopkins University where he taught pharmacology and where he also established department of clinical pharmacology, the first one in the world. In 1970 he became the first chairman of the Department of Pharmacology and Toxicology at the University of Rochester where he founded the Center for Study of Drug Development.[116] Fourteen years later Dr. Lasagna moved along with the Center to Tufts University in Boston and became dean of the Sackler School of Graduate Biomedical Sciences. Dr. Lasagna dedicated his life to medicine and ethical rules in clinical research and medical ethics in general and never forgot to emphasize how high cost of medical education works to the public's disadvantage because it reduces the talent pool to people from top range of socio-economic scale.

Dr. Lasagna wrote in The Times Magazine in 1964 that 'the new doctor has lost a sense of continuity with the past without gaining a bond with his contemporaries' and called for a worldwide competition for an updated Hippocratic Oath. In his own words 'warmth, sympathy and understanding may outweigh the surgeon's knife or chemist's drug.' It is still read at some medical school graduation ceremonies.[117]

---

[116]   KI Kaitian. 2003. "A Tribute to Dr.Louis C. Lasagna: 1923-2003." *Drug Information Journal* 37: 353–54.

[117]   Nora Krug. "Louis Lasagna, 80, a Doctor and an Expert on Placebos, Dies." *The New York Times*.

Over his lifetime Dr. Lasagna wrote or co-authored 655 academic papers[118] and two popular books 'The Doctors' Dilemma' (1962) and 'Life, Death and the Doctor' (1968). His most widely recognized works related to the response to placebo which he believed is dependent on psychosomatic type of the patient rather than effect of the drug. Lasagna's team at the Massachusetts General Hospital in Boston was the first to investigate placebo and how patients who respond positively to placebo differ from those who do not. In their most cited paper 'A Study of the Placebo Response' they studied post-operative pain in 162 patients who underwent general, gynecologic, orthopedic, or urologic surgery. Of sixty-nine patients who received at least two placebo injections instead of real painkillers the doctors evaluated the consistency of the placebo response and found out that 16% patients consistently positively responded to placebo, 29% consistently did not respond, and 55% patients showed inconsistent reaction. After this the evaluated the study participants psychologically through a series of various psychometric tests and found out that responders and non-responders differ in many significant ways. They also concluded that responders and non-responders can be revealed by a series of tests and intense interviews but not by quick assessments and impression they make on staff. In total, Henry K Beecher and Louis Lasagna conducted series of studies in which they identified 1,082 patients who consistently positively responded to placebo.[119]

In the book 'Doctor's Dilemmas' (1962) Lasagna described controversy which revolves around the risk attendant on the early evaluation of new drugs. Many clinical investigators rightly resent running risks of malpractice litigation following accidents with experimental drugs and are not eager to experiment at their own peril. They (the physicians) want the industry to shoulder some of the responsibility and to at least sit down and discuss the

---

[118] "Louis C. Lasagna Papers (1947-2001)." 2014. River Campus Libraries at University of Rochester: Department of rare books, special collections, and preservation.

[119] S Scheindlin. 2009. "The Problematic Placebo. Reflections: Science in Cultural Context." *Molecular Interventions* 9 (3): 108–13.

malpractice coverage problem as it pertains to the investigators collecting the data for a pharmaceutical firm.[120]

In 1968, Louis Lasagna published his second book *'Life, Death, and the Doctor'* in which he is very critical of physicians who fall into a comfortable routine without any need to upgrade their education and keep up with advances in medicine, and fail to find balance between long hours of well-paid medical practice and costly self-improvement. He discussed lack of uniformed standards in medical licensing from one part of the country to another and the need to maintain medical standards for all practitioners. In this book, but also in countless short works and presentations he had at medical schools, he stressed problems of that time such as medical experimentation on humans, world population explosion, birth control, abortion, aging, end of life medicine, and the need to assess epidemiological risks of the effect of atmospheric pollutants and the demand for realistic standards and controls.

Lasagna paid special attention to the patient-doctor contract, controversies relating to medical care provided to the poor, patients' autonomy and the informed consent, professional confidences, testimonies provided by doctors in court, legal restraints imposed on patients afflicted with insanity, and difficulties which medical science has when confronted with legal aspects of drug abuse and the whole philosophy of the law with regards to drug abuse.[121]

Lasagna was a consultant to the Food and Drug Administration and many other organizations in the USA and abroad, most importantly as a chairman of the President's National Committee to Review Current Procedures for Approval of New Drugs for Cancer and AIDS, and member of the Blue Ribbon Panel which was established to assess FDA performance and recommend initiatives aimed to improve effectiveness of the Agency. Lasagna's contribution had crucial impact on the way clinical trials are conducted today. He

---

[120]   Lasagna, L: Doctor's Dilemmas. NY: Harper & Row, 1962.

[121]   H Wing. 1969. "Louis Lasagna, Life, Death, and the Doctor." *Valparaiso University Law Review* 3 (2, Art 11): 318–20.

was an outspoken advocate of stricter rules on drug approvals and promoted randomized controlled trials as the golden standard.[122] Lasagna testified before the U.S. Congress many times, most importantly at the 1962 Kefauver hearings, which led to implementation of new requirements for the assessment of effectiveness of new drugs.[123]

The Kefauver-Harris Amendment of 1962 was a reaction to the infamous thalidomide affair which fundamentally changed rules for new drug development. The 1938 Food, Drug, & Cosmetics Act had serious shortcomings, like e.g. manufacturers could place a new drug on the market if the FDA failed to respond within 60 days. In addition to that, FDA had no authority to enforce good manufacturing practices. By 1962, the real effects of hypnotic thalidomide became known and it was clear that a change in market regulation is long overdue. Thalidomide was first approved as a sedative for over-the-counter sales in West Germany in 1953 as a drug which was allegedly completely non-toxic. Rats on which the drug was tested failed to fall asleep but were less active. Brief tests on people showed that the drug did have hypnotic effect on people.

The wonder drug was approved for insomnia, coughs, colds, and headaches, and morning sickness which frequently troubled pregnant women. By 1961, Grünenthal managed to obtain approval in forty-six countries. First complaints regarding potential toxicity of thalidomide appeared in scientific journals in 1959 when peripheral neuropathy was reported in long-term users of thalidomide but Grünenthal did all it could first to hide the evidence and later to play down the side effects, and in 1960 attempted to enter the U.S. market. The firm's research director Heinrich Mückter lost confidence in safety of thalidomide as the evidence was accumulating. In 1961, obstetricians William McBride (Australian) and Widukind Lenz (German) voiced a suspicion there was a link between birth defects and thalidomide use in early stage

---

[122] JH Tanne. 2003. "Louis Lasagna." *BMJ* 327 (7414): 565.

[123] Nora Krug. "Louis Lasagna, 80, a Doctor and an Expert on Placebos, Dies." *The New York Times.*

of pregnancy.[124]

In August 1961, Germany restricted thalidomide sales to prescription only and Grünenthal reluctantly removed 'nontoxic' from the label. But the worst was still to come. Pregnant women were often prescribed thalidomide for morning sickness. A year after introduction of thalidomide, first babies with missing limbs were born. Whilst this deformity under normal circumstances is very rare, after introduction of thalidomide its incidence increased two-hundred times. Dr. Lenz was the first one who associated these otherwise rare birth defects with thalidomide taken in early pregnancy and published his observation in German press. Although Grünenthal accused Dr. Lenz of spreading a rumor with the intent to kill the drug, in November 1961 the firm finally halted thalidomide sales in Germany; however, it continued selling the drug abroad until January 1963. By then, 13,000 babies were born with missing limbs.[125]

Thalidomide was first licensed in the UK in 1958 by Distillers Biochemical Ltd (currently Diageo), a company which normally dealt with liquor and desired to establish itself on the market with sedatives and hypnotics. Ten years later, the company reached compensation settlement with affected families. Victims of thalidomide in Germany were not that lucky because many of them only received compensation decades later. Grünenthal only officially apologized in September 2012.[126] One of the families affected by thalidomide commented on this late apology:

> *'Our family couldn't have gone into silent shock. We had to get up and face each day and every day and cope with the incredible damage that Gruenenthal drug did to Lyn and our family.'*

---

[124] News Medical. 2014. "History of Thalidomide." *News Medical.*

[125] Ellen Rice. 2007. "Dr. Frances Kelsey: Turning the Thalidomide Tragedy into Food and Drug Administration Reform."

[126] C Mackenzie. 2012. "German Firm Which Invented Birth Defect Drug Thalidomide Apologizes for the First Time in 50 Years - but British Charity Demands Compensation." *Daily Mail.*

Limbless victims of a 'harmless drug' which was in fact teratogenic had to cope with ever increasing costs of care with no financial help from the firm which directly caused their disability. None of the corporate executives was ever prosecuted.[127]

Only after series of deaths from an untested formulation of Elixir Sulfonamide in 1937 laws on pre-marketing drug testing were implemented. In 1960, FDA had no right to require proof of safety and efficacy of newly approved drugs, and there were no regulations regarding the way drugs were tested before marketing. Because it was the drug-makers, who controlled the testing, to whom all the test data belonged, and which were effectively preventing the authorities from access to it, clinical experiments could be performed without the FDA's knowledge and consent. Americans were spared the thalidomide disaster not due to strength of their agency and their laws but due to vigilance of one woman who got this application for approval on her desk.

Novice FDA investigator, Dr. Frances Oldham Kelsey, refused to approve the drug on the U.S. market because she was concerned about its potential for teratogenic effects. This attitude was by no means common within the FDA. At that time, FDA doctors wrote promotional articles in scientific journals on new drugs, and FDA investigators were ordered by officials to certify new drugs based on company data because the company itself was the best judge of its safety. In this sense, Dr. Kelsey went directly against the FDA policy and fortunately for her, found backup both in the FDA and in academia before it was taken to Congress. Kelsey's demand for proof of safety of thalidomide came at the right time and led to series of Congressional hearings and implementation of the Kefauver-Harris amendment[128] and eventually to profound reform of the Food and Drug Administration in which Dr. Louis Lasagna directly participated in terms of definition of design of clinical trials. The most important authorities given to FDA by the

---

[127]   Reuters. 2014. "Thalidomide Inventors Apologize for Birth Defects, 50 Years Later."

[128]   FDA. 2014. "Kefauver-Harris Amendments Revolutionized Drug Development."

Kefauver-Harris Amendment were that manufacturers were from now on required to prove effectiveness based on adequate and well-controlled clinical studies and conducted by qualified experts on subjects who provided informed consent with drug testing before market launch and report serious side effects. The amendment gave FDA the authority to retrospectively evaluate safety of drugs approved in the period between 1938 and 1962, and allowed FDA to set good manufacturing standards for industry and conduct inspections.[129]

Louis Lasagna was the initiator of one of the most important amendments of rules for clinical experiments and won numerous honors and awards over his lifetime. The 'Father of clinical pharmacology' as he was called died n August 2003. Among all these lifelong achievements, he wrote modernized version of Hippocratic Oath which is in use by many medical schools today at graduation ceremonies:

> I swear to fulfill, to the best of my ability and judgment, this covenant:
>
> I will respect the hard-won scientific gains of those physicians in whose steps I walk, and gladly share such knowledge as is mine with those who are to follow.
>
> I will apply, for the benefit of the sick, all measures [that] are required, avoiding those twin traps of overtreatment and therapeutic nihilism.
>
> I will remember that there is art to medicine as well as science, and that warmth, sympathy, and understanding may outweigh the surgeon's knife or the chemist's drug.
>
> I will not be ashamed to say "I know not," nor will I fail to call in my colleagues when the skills of another are needed for a patient's recovery.
>
> I will respect the privacy of my patients, for their problems are not disclosed to me that the world may know.

---

[129]   LA Seidman, and N Warren. 2001. "Educating the Biotechnology Workforce: Pharmaceutical Regulation in the United States." *Biolink*.

Most especially must I tread with care in matters of life and death. If it is given me to save a life, all thanks. But it may also be within my power to take a life; this awesome responsibility must be faced with great humbleness and awareness of my own frailty. Above all, I must not play at God.

I will remember that I do not treat a fever chart, a cancerous growth, but a sick human being, whose illness may affect the person's family and economic stability. My responsibility includes these related problems, if I am to care adequately for the sick.

I will prevent disease whenever I can, for prevention is preferable to cure.

I will remember that I remain a member of society, with special obligations to all my fellow human beings those sound of mind and body as well as the infirm.

If I do not violate this oath, may I enjoy life and art, respected while I live and remembered with affection thereafter. May I always act so as to preserve the finest traditions of my calling and may I long experience the joy of healing those who seek my help.

SOVIET MEDICAL OATH

The Supreme Soviet approved medical oath of the USSR in 1971. Just like the Nazi Gesundheit, Soviet medical oath prioritized strongly interests of society, Soviet state, and mankind as a whole to the interests of individual patients. Soviet physicians were obliged to work to aid the development of medical science and follow the guidance of Communist morality. In 1983 the clause on prevention of nuclear war was added to the oath. Upon having conferred on me the high calling of physician and entering medical practice, I do solemnly swear:

> To dedicate all my knowledge and strength to the preservation and improvement of the health of mankind and to the treatment and prevention of disease, and to work in good conscience wherever it is required by society;
>
> To be always ready to provide medical care, to relate to the patient attentively and carefully, and to preserve medical confidences;
>
> To constantly perfect my medical knowledge and clinical skills and thereby in my work to aid in the development of medical science and practice;
>
> To refer, if the patient's better interests warrant it, for advice from my fellow physicians, and never myself to refuse to give such advice or help;
>
> To preserve and develop the noble traditions of Soviet medicine, to be guided in all my actions by the principles of Communist morality, and to always bear in mind the high calling of a Soviet physician and my responsibility to the people and to the Soviet state.
>
> Recognizing the danger which nuclear weaponry presents for mankind, I promise to struggle tirelessly for peace and for the prevention of nuclear war. I swear to be loyal to this oath as long as I live. [130]

---

[130] "Physician Oaths." 2014. American Association of Physicians and Surgeons.

Practical implementation of Soviet Oath

Soviet medicine did not follow the same development as medical science in the West. Soviet Union was the first country in the world to grant every citizen "constitutional right to health" in the sense of "right to health-care" already in 1917. This right did not affect numbers of casualties of First and Second World Wars which were the highest of all participating countries, both in absolute and relative numbers. Apart from troubles to catch up with western standards, Soviet medicine manifested some very specific differences which were unique to the Communist Block.

History of experiments on human subjects directly ordered by the government starts in the 1920's in 'Laboratory 12' run by Soviet NKVD. In this laboratory, the Soviets were testing lethal poisons on 'Enemies of the People'. Evidence relating to this top secret facility was only discovered in the early 1990's when several researchers managed to obtain secret documents and testimonies from people who decided to talk when the regime fell. The first laboratory was directly established by Lenin already in 1921 and delegated to Professor Ignaty Kazakov who remained in charge of the facility until 1938.

Before the Great War the laboratory was taken over by Boris Zbarsky, a scientist from the Department of Biochemistry and Analytical Chemistry at the First Moscow Medical Institute. Several scientists from the Bach Institute of Biochemistry directly participated in the same program. Zbarsky mainly specialized in narcotics and their administration, and throughout his career he managed to maintain excellent relationships with both Felix Dzierzhinskii and his successor Genrikh Yagoda. Kazakov and Yagoda were accused by new head of the NKVD Ezhov of establishing a poison laboratory, which was true, and of preparing a sinister plot to poison Ezhov, which was not, but it did not matter as they both were executed after a show trial to make sure they do not get any ideas. Senior Major of State Security S.B. Zhukovskii was appointed as the Head of the Administrative-Economic Department which supervised secret poisons laboratory since

October 1936.[131] Ezhov was appointed head of NKVD in November 1936. In summer 1938, the State Security Department was reorganized and the poison laboratory was moved from 12th Department to 2nd Special Department which otherwise dealt with operational equipment.

Mikhail Alyokhin was appointed an acting head in summer 1938. Zhukovskii was arrested on May 3, 1939, and testified that the poison laboratory was headed by sadist biochemist Grigory Marianovskii, better known as Doctor Death, and engineer Arkady Osinkin, who worked with Ezhov's first deputy M.P. Frinovskii, his own deputy Mikhail Alyokhin, and Major of State Security V.S. Tsesarskii, Head of the 1st Special Section which was in charge of especially sensitive operations; and its main purpose was to prepare poisons to be used in terror campaigns against Soviet leaders. Alyokhin was fired in a few weeks for being a 'German spy', and succeeded by Yevgeny Lapshin, Arkady Osinkin, and Valentin Kravchenko.

In February 1939 the department was split in two and expanded: Lapshin's 2nd Special Department now had 621 staff, whilst the 4th Special Department headed by Mikhail Filimonov was ten times smaller. It became known as the Laboratory No. 1 or the 'Kamera' (Chamber); and it was intended and used for testing of products invented by chemical laboratory supervised by Mairanovsky, and biological laboratory supervised by Sergei Muromtsev. The experimental subjects were provided by Vasily Blokhin, chief NKVD executioner, from Lubyanka and Butyrka prisons. Ezhov was succeeded by Lavrenty Beria in November 1938. During the interrogation which took place in May and June 1939, Zhukovskii tried to shift the blame for poison operations to Ezhov, Frinovskii, and Alyokhin, whilst Ezhov and others were blaming Zhukovskii. All four were condemned to death and executed in January 1940.

Maironovskii was too valuable scientist to be shot and was allowed to survive. His original tests with yperite were disappointing

---

[131]   M Parish. *Sacrifice of the Generals: Soviet Senior Officer Losses, 1939-1953; Pp 97-100.* Scarecrow Press, Inc.

because the cause of death was immediately obvious during autopsies. This was not what Miranovsky tried to achieve as his main objective was to find a poison which would be organoleptically undetectable and which would not leave trace after death. Substance K-2, chemically carbylamines choline-chloride, had all desired properties and killed its victims in fifteen minutes. He also experimented with ricin, digitoxin, and curare. His followers continued testing various poisons, hypnotism techniques, and interrogation techniques on living people until 1953[132].

According to Sudoplatov, Maironovskii was the one who ordered Abakumov to arrange the killing of Wallenberg.[133] Mairanovsky was eventually arrested in 1951 and sentenced to ten years in prison. During his investigation Filimonov testified that Sudoplatov and Eitingon would not approve special equipment, meaning poisons intended for actual use for assassinations, without testing them on humans. As he said, some of these poisons caused extreme suffering to the victims. The laboratory itself was officially closed down but in fact moved to the Department of Special Equipment. Its research continues to be exploited by the State Security.

In 1953, former Trotsky's secretary Wolfgang Salus was assassinated by an MGB agent Otto Freitag who gave him a special substance which caused pneumonia-like symptoms. Salus died in one of Munich's hospitals without anyone noticing anything out of the ordinary. In the 1950's and 1960's, the products of the Special Laboratory called Lab X headed by Vladimir Naumov were used against enemies of the people in exile. Nikolai Khokhlov, a failed assassin who instead of killing his target turned himself in and became cooperator of the FBI, was in 1957 poisoned by radioactive thallium. He was lucky to get in the U.S. Army medical facility where his condition was promptly diagnosed. Khokhlov survived, in the difference from Litvinenko who was poisoned by radioactive polonium 210 five decades later. Ukrainian émigrés Lev Rebet and

---

[132]   Boris Volodarsky. 2009. *The KGB's Poison Factory from Lenin to Litvinenko*, *pp 32-48*. Frontline Books. Zenith Press.

[133]   M Parrish. *Sacrifice of the Generals: Soviet Senior Officer Losses, 1939-1953*; *Pp 97-100*. Scarecrow Press, Inc.

Stepan Bandera were both poisoned by Russian operative Bogdan Stashinsky in 1959.[134] After serving 8 years in prison, Stashinsky was given very substantial assistance with resettlement in exchange for sharing information on political assassinations with western agencies.

In 1978, Laboratory 12 was reorganized again. It became part of Operational Technical Directorate of the KGB under revised name Central Scientific Research Institute for Special Technology. A year after signing the Biological and Toxin Weapons Convention, Biopreparat was established under the cover of Pharmaceutical and Vaccine Company. Biopreparat, massive complex of some forty facilities, was in charge of research and production of biological weapons, where 25 to 32,000 employees were working on development of new weapons and cures and antidotes against them. Additional 10,000 Ministry of Defense staff worked in bioweapons laboratories. This information was brought to the West after 1989 mainly by Vladimir Pasechnik, Dr Kanatjan Alibekov, and Dr Vil Mirzayanov. According to General Nikolai Golushko, current scientific and technological directorate carries out operations with the sanctions of the procurator and in compliance with the Constitution and the courts.

In September 2004, Ukrainian presidential candidate Vladimir Yushchenko fell gravely ill after eating dioxine-enriched dinner. Two years later, in November 2006, Russian defector Alexander Litvinenko was fatally poisoned with polonium 210. Both cases made headlines and were extensively reported in world media. Other poisons used by Soviet doctors were labeled as 'soft' chemicals which were only designed for interrogation purposes. SP-17, a truth drug, was one of them. Another one, 'Injection C', caused the victims to become extremely talkative and willing to answer any questions asked before they died. Death followed in about twenty-four hours. 'Soft' chemicals were used for temporary incapacitation of the target.[135]

---

[134]   Boris Volodarsky. *The KGB's Poison Factory from Lenin to Litvinenko*, Frontline Books. Zenith Press 2009.

[135]   Ibid.

Leon Trotsky's son Leon Sedov became victim to medical foul play on French territory when in exile. The NKVD surveillance team followed Sedov and his associates at all times for several years. One of them, Renate Steiner, befriended Sedov and his mistress Jeanne Martin and spent most of the time on vacations with the couple. Sedov was not suspicious about her at all and thought she was a pleasant, timid, young, and insignificant female. Renate later testified in court with regards to Sedov's murder and mentioned Efron as the agent who was responsible for preparation of Sedov's assassination. Sedov was getting ready for a trip to Mulhouse with great secrecy but the NKVD was prepared for him and awaited him there. Shortly before leaving, Sedov suddenly canceled the trip because of alleged ill health. This information came from Lilia and the illness was also mentioned in Etienne's letter to Trotsky. Jeanne Martin, Sedov's mistress, was telling a different story: according to her, Leon Sedov was in good shape and enjoyed excellent health; and was very resilient mentally as well. In her testimony she stated that Sedov fell ill suddenly on January 15, and was diagnosed with appendicitis; but was well again five days later. Abdominal pains recurred two weeks later, and he was admitted to the Mirabeau Clinic, a small Russian hospital owned and directed by Boris Zhimursky.

The decision to take him to this facility was made by Jeanne, Lilia, and Dr. Trachtenberg, Lilia's sister-in-law in an apparent belief that 'there were no Russians in the hospital'. In the meantime, Etienne arranged transport by an ambulance whilst Lilia went for money needed for hospitalization. The NKVD team was watching the whole scene from the opposite building in rue Lacratelle. Sedov was hospitalized under the name Monsieur Martin in order to hide his identity. Zhimursky, according to the the police a Bolshevik sympathizer, came from Russia in 1928 with enough money to sustain both high standard of living and to open a hospital in Paris. Dr Simkov, graduate from Geneva Medical School, became director of Zhimursky's clinic in 1931. He, too, was pro-Soviet. Lilia denied knowledge of this and convinced Trotsky that both doctors are apolitical. In addition to that, her friend, Dr. Faum Trachtenberg, initially took care of Sedov despite having no license to practice.

There was only one nurse of Russian origin working in the hospital: Helena Eismond, and she took care of Sedov more often than any other nurse. The only doctor who was aware of Sedov's true identity was Dr. Trachtenberg. In reality it would have been much safer if the hospital was French and if the doctors were told his true identity. Dr. Marcel Thalheimer was the only medic who was not listed as Russian. He operated Sedov twice, the first time successfully on February 9 when he allegedly removed an 'intestinal occlusion', and the second time, five days later when his condition suddenly and unexpectedly deteriorated. While Etienne and Lilia thought Sedov died naturally of post-operational complications, Jeanne Martin was convinced that there was foul play involved in sudden worsening of his state during the night 13-14th February, and with the help of lawyers Jean Rous, Gerard Rosenthal and Sedov's father Leon Trotsky, she managed to obtain original post-mortem investigation and statements. Dr. Thalheimer was unable to explain the sudden crisis and opted for re-operation because of suspected auto-intoxication, but the patient died the following day. At that time, Lilia wrote a letter to Trotsky in which she mentioned Sedov's alleged constant ill health through 1937, and Jeanne's neurasthenic lunatic imaginations about foul play in an apparent attempt to prove that Sedov's death was a natural one. The official version was that the patient jumped out of his bed at night, walked to a different room, found an orange and ate it, and fell on a bed in the other room where he was later found. The hospital refused to identify the patients who witnessed the incident. Jeanne remembered that the fateful morning on February 14th Sedov said 'You know what they did to me last night' but was too weak to explain what happened to him. There was a purple patch on his abdomen that morning and Jeanne suspected poisoning. There were four inquiries into his death in total, but most of them turned out to be mere formality which failed to produce anything of substance. In the difference from Jeanne, Trotsky eventually accepted the verdict that Sedov's death was natural one, and stopped communicating with her because further investigations would have threatened their immigration status in France.[136]

---

[136]   RT Kronenbitter. 2014. "Leon Trotsky, Dupe of the NKVD. How the Soviets Destroyed the Fourth International." *CIA Library – Center for the Study of Intelligence.*

But ordinary well-behaved Soviet citizens were not spared of advances of socialistic medicine either. In 1986, specialist in pulmonary medicine from Columbia College of Physicians, and Surgeons in New York, Dr Kenneth M Prager privately visited Moscow and Leningrad, and wrote a detailed article about his experience which was published in the Wall Street Journal. Dr Prager wrote that Soviet medical-care system is decades behind the West in technology that can adequately care for simple ailments, and offers bathing in mineral waters in Spa resorts in lieu of medical care.

Most astonishingly, Soviet system cares very poorly for its own veterans who have to wait long time for wheelchairs and whose prosthetic devices are very primitive. Surgical gloves and other disposable items are washed and reused; and sterilization is done by boiling the items in water. Advances in pharmacotherapy completely missed Soviet territory, and new medications are either unavailable or so scarce that their use in the treatment of chronic diseases becomes meaningless. Extreme shortages include medications such as cimetidine, beta-blockers, calcium channel inhibitors, or antihistamines.

Low quality of birth-control results in high numbers of abortions. According to conservative Soviet statistics, Soviet woman undergoes six abortions in her lifetime, and it is not uncommon to see a woman who had 10 or 15. Even though the health care is in theory free, few people dare to rely on it and bring a roll of rubles with them to make sure they get their linen changed and receive their medication. Their families have to bring them food from home. Starvation diets are commonly prescribed to treat chronic illness. In this classless society, some citizens are more equal than others. These flagships of Soviet medicine which are intended for Communist Party leaders and other prominent figures are the only hospitals which an unsuspecting foreigner is likely to see.[137] If ordinary Soviet citizens did not get much out of the system without

---

[137]   Prager KM. 1987. "Soviet Health Care's Critical Condition." *The Wall Street Journal*, January 29.

extra payments, enemies of the people were getting even rougher deal. Not only they were unlikely to receive adequate treatment when needed even if they were able to afford to pay for it, which they were typically not; they were often systematically harmed by denial of health care and rough living conditions caused by paralyzing poverty or life in various institutions and prisons.

MEDICAL OATHS USED TODAY

In 1993, a large-scale study of the oaths administered by almost 150 North American medical schools was undertaken to determine the popularity and content of modern oaths. Oath-taking upon graduation is very popular, and practiced by nearly all medical schools. Eighty years ago, less than one quarter of doctors-to-be took an oath. The atrocities of Second World War dramatically increased the popularity of oath-taking and the popular demand for formal implementation of ethical rules for physicians. Some oaths are entirely separate from legal obligations of physicians, whilst others directly refer to valid legislation in the text of the oath. Original Hippocratic Oath was a legally binding act. Today, it mainly shows determination to act ethically, and to continue lifelong self-education. After the Second World War, many medical schools started using the World Medical Association Oath, just to return to the spirit of Hippocrates later on. Some medical schools modified Hippocratic Oath and created their own versions; others adopted the Lasagna Oath as a modernized version of Hippocratic Oath.

Controversial topics such as abortions and euthanasia were often omitted not to create conflict for the physician. In early 1970's, as a result of series of affairs such as the Tuskegee syphilis study or experiments with radioisotopes and epidemiologic studies performed on people who were living in dangerous areas such as nuclear dump-sites without being informed about this fact, led to widespread interest in bioethics. American Hospital Association adopted the Patient's Bill of Rights, the Belmont Report, the National Research Act, and the foundation of the Kennedy Institute of Ethics. Two landmark cases changed the medical oaths in the USA because the Supreme Court expressed opinion on two fundamental topics which were part of the Hippocratic Oath: abortion and euthanasia. Ban on abortion and providing a client with a deadly poison is common to all ancient medical oaths. In the case Roe vs. Wade the Supreme Court in 1973 decided in favor of performing an abortion. The case effectively caused split in public opinion in two major camps: pro-choice in favor of abortions as woman's right for privacy as defined in the 14th Amendment of the U.S. Constitution; and pro-life, in favor of the right of the unborn to life. The Karen Ann Quinlan case which appeared in front of the U.S. Supreme Court in 1976 decided in favor of active intervention toward a patient's death, and effectively granted the patient the right to die by allowing the doctors to remove her from a respirator. These two Supreme Court decisions initiated series of revisions of medical oaths in the United States toward omission of the clause on ban on abortions and ban on euthanasia.

INDIAN MEDICAL OATHS

Most medical oaths used in India today originate in the West, although modifications of versions of Hippocratic Oath currently in use reflect Indian culture. This revised version by Pai and Pandy includes the duty of a physician first to take into consideration patient's welfare; refers to the heritage of Charaka and Suhruta; and as the only medical oath in the world also includes commitment of a newly graduating physician to participate in teaching and research as well as medical practice. Care for patients with incurable diseases emphasizes patient's welfare which means palliative treatment over patient's survival.

> *"On this day, as I graduate as a physician, I take this oath. I shall practice the art and science of medicine honestly, sincerely and to the best of my ability and judgment. I understand the responsibility that the profession entails. The patient's welfare will be central to all my activities. I shall honor the rich heritage of ethics that we have inherited from Charaka, Sushruta and other great Indian teachers of the past. I shall do my best to participate in all three facets of medical practice: care of patients, research and teaching."*

> *"I will care for my patients in a scientific and ethical manner. I will provide the best of care to all my patients without any consideration of their religion, caste, personal beliefs or socioeconomic status. In those patients where cure is impossible I shall attempt to relieve pain and suffering. I will continue to offer my care and concern to the end. Above all, I will do nothing that may harm the patient."*

This commitment to treat all patients equally regardless their economic standing was not part of the original Hippocratic Oath. Although it did emphasize compassion it did not expect the physician to treat all the poor who were unable to afford to pay for his services at the expense of those who were more affluent. The Oath of American Medical Association went much further than that, and heavily regulated any free consultations and treatments provided to the poor. This statement in the Indian Oath directly relates to the whole concept of prioritizing patient's welfare rather than cure, and palliative care for patients with 'incurable' diseases who are only required to receive pain relief and comfort till the end.

> *"Medical science keeps improving and learning is a life-long process. I shall continue reading learned journals and attend continuing education programs. I will do my best to be conversant with recent advances and new thinking in medicine. Thus I will keep improving the care of my patients."*

Requirement of continuous education is not explicitly mentioned in most medical oaths. The next section is also very interesting because it allows exceptions for disclosure of medical secrets when directed by law.

> *"I shall respect and maintain my patients' secrets. Where required, with the patient's permission, I shall also take into confidence the family, so that my patient gets the best treatment possible. There will be occasions when, in the greater interests of society, I am required by law to divulge confidential information. I will do all I can to ensure that my patient's interests are protected and that the need for making confidential information public is known to my patient."*

Other medical oaths usually describe best practice rather than listing possible malpractice. Commission offered by a service provider shall not be taken by the practitioner because such practice would be unethical, and would unnecessarily burden the patient.

> *"I will not perform needless investigations or procedures that are unlikely to benefit my patient. I neither expect nor will I accept payment from my colleagues, laboratories, imaging institutes or any other organization, offered as commission or share of their income. I shall practice only the specialty in which I have training. I am aware of my limitations. There will be times when my patient needs the help of someone wiser, more knowledgeable or skilled. I shall have no hesitation in requesting such help. Should the patient request a second opinion, I will help in obtaining it."*

Indian medical oath also acknowledges other medical schools, especially traditional Ayurveda, and imposes sharp divide between. Physicians trained and certified in modern medicine are not allowed to use in their practice methods and medicines they were not trained in.

> *"I shall restrict my practice to modern medicine, in which I have been trained. I shall not use drugs or preparations from other branches of medicine unless I am trained in their use and am certified to use them."*

As the only medical oath, Indian version encourages research in medicine as beneficial to others providing the patient is well-informed and understands the inquiry. The same applies to presentation of own research at conferences, publication activity, and dedication to teaching. Other medical oaths do not emphasize this component of medical practice as compulsory part of the 'doctor's life mission'.

> *"My research will depend on my circumstances but my enquiring spirit will search for problems, the solutions to which will benefit patients. Just as I would not like to be treated as a guinea pig, I will ensure that my patients participate in my studies as well-informed individuals, fully conversant with the purpose of the enquiry, the questions asked, answers sought and how these may benefit others. All my dealings will be honest and transparent. I shall endeavor to teach my younger or less experienced colleagues what I have learnt in medicine. I will do my best to pass on the fruits of my education and experience to my patients and to my colleagues through the media, and papers presented at conferences and published in medical journals."*

The last section of the modern Indian medical oath contains yet another clause on bribery and marketing tactics of other professions, pharmaceutical companies, and insurers. Care for a patient shall not be compromised by business interests of the physician. Respect to teachers and treating colleagues with courtesy and consideration is then part of all other medical oaths, and the Indian one is no exception in this.

"Whilst I understand the need for drug companies to market their products, I shall not make myself their tool and shall be careful not to allow my judgment to be affected by their sales tactics. My dealings with their representatives will be courteous but transparent. Because healthcare often involves multiple professions, including insurance companies and other agencies, I shall interact with the members of other related professions in a correct manner such that the care of the patient is not compromised in any way."

"I believe that my work will speak for itself. Advertisement in any manner is beneath the dignity of my profession. In keeping with Indian tradition, I will continue to respect and be grateful to all my teachers. I shall treat all my colleagues with courtesy. I cherish the wisdom in the teaching that lies in the Golden Rule. I will do for my patient everything I would expect my doctor to do for me, were I the patient."[138]

Oath of Indian Medical Association

I solemnly pledge myself to consecrate my life to service of humanity.

Even under threat, I will not use my medical knowledge contrary to the laws of Humanity.

I will maintain the utmost respect for human life from the time of conception.

I will not permit considerations of religion, nationality, race, party politics or social standing to intervene between my duty and my patient.

I will practice my profession with conscience and dignity.

The health of my patient will be my first consideration.

I will respect the secrets which are confined in me.

I will give to my teachers the respect and gratitude which is their due.

---

[138] SA Pai, and SK Pandya. 2010. "Speaking for Ourselves. A Revised Hippocratic Oath for Indian Medical Students." *The National Medical Journal of India* 23 (6): 360–61.

I will maintain by all means in my power, the honor and noble traditions of medical profession.

I will treat my colleagues with all respect and dignity.

I shall abide by the code of medical ethics as enunciated in the Indian Medical Council (Professional Conduct, Etiquette and Ethics) Regulations 2002.

I make these promises solemnly, freely and upon my honor.

This last medical oath is given to medical students to sign at registration with the Indian Medical Association. It directly refers to regulations which the practitioner is supposed to follow. Oath-taking in many professions is a form of introduction in the profession. It depends on culture how seriously is an act like that taken. Its meaning varies from a text of mostly historical and emotional value to a sacred act which binds the person for life to a special profession. It is not a universal document, and from its very nature it can never be the same all over the globe, because the differences in understanding human nature and the role of a physician in society are simply too great. When doctors move from one country to another, they generally do not retake a medical oath, but only have to get their qualifications and certification recognized or updated to align themselves with local requirements. In a host country, doctors are supposed to follow the regulations of a country they practice in. In the era of Hippocrates, medical oath was a legally binding document which was also enforceable in real time. This has fundamentally changed as there are other mechanisms which replaced medical oath as a legal document. Medical oath only serves as a reminder of special role of medical profession, and the duty of every single physician to live up to the expectations, and not to abuse the art and knowledge he or she acquired.

IV. THE EUGENIC TRAIL

To be from a 'good family' has always been an advantage in access to power and opportunities in life because people with favorable historical record within society would be generally accepted better by the community as 'worth the investment', no matter what the definition of 'favorable characteristics' would be. In the late 19th century, eugenics became a widely accepted discipline in the medical community. Its scientific rationale made its way to other parts of societal and public life, including law enforcement. In the quest for causes of crime, people's background was extensively scrutinized in efforts to find characteristics which would allow detection of would-be criminals before they have a chance to commit an actual 'crime'. According to popular theories of that time pauperism and inclination toward asocial behavior were perceived as hereditary traits. Formulation of these thoughts by contemporary authors coincides with the emergence of Darwin's evolutionary theory, which is used as basis for these works. Techniques known from animal husbandry, as well as and experience with breeding of domestic animals, were extrapolated to human population in the same way. The most prolific works of that time are the writings of Francis Galton, whose 'Hereditary Genius' is essentially a case for the superiority of genetic material of well-established British noble families, and defense of their claim to power. While it is possible that the main motivation was simply to promote theory of his cousin Charles Darwin, the historical context which has to be taken into consideration suggests that the main motivation could be the uneasy relationship between Britain and France, and the threat of spread of the '1848 French troubles' to the British Monarchy.

THE NOBLE CAUSE

Eugenic movement started in Britain. Although there is little consensus among historians what facilitated its spread and wide acceptance; it is safe to assume that political turmoil in years after the French revolution would have caused widespread efforts within then elite to push back against similar movements at home, and provide scientific evidence which would justify hereditary entitlement of the contemporary elite to power. As the eugenic movement was picking up speed in the U.S., other motivations were contributing to the widespread acceptance of these theories. U.S. Bill of Rights as ratified in December 1791 acknowledged many rights to all U.S. citizens which were at that time not codified in European monarchies.

Eugenics only spread to America in the end of 19th century, mainly after the 1892 International Congress on Demographics in London where Galton presented his research and his books. Galton's Hereditary Genius was published in New York the same year. Even though there were state laws prohibiting intimate contact between blacks and the majority white population, American eugenics was primarily directed against 'paupers', 'ne'er-do-wells', and 'morons', in attempts to enhance quality of its population, and efforts to find the root cause of criminal and asocial behavior.

Study 'The Jukes' (1874) describes how much public resources had to be spent on numerous descendants of a poor white family, and how little they contributed to society over generations. Similar studies, such as Davenport's research efforts, wide access of protagonists of eugenics to various conferences, together with widespread acceptance of eugenics as a concept by the scientific community, as well as the general public, caused that very few objections were raised when Indiana sterilization law was enacted.

When the Nuremberg laws were implemented in Germany in 1933-35, the world did not object mainly because the concept itself was not perceived as fundamentally wrong at that time. Only as time went it became obvious that Nazi Germany is going to turn the announced 'invigoration' of their nation into a killing machine. Eugenic movement provided all the evidence and reasoning necessary for Hitler to write his Mein Kampf, formulate Nazi medical oath (Gesundheit) and build the whole system of systematic disposal of 'low value' human stock.

BACK TO THE TRIBE OF LEVI

The Book of Leviticus is the third book of the Hebrew Bible, and the third of five books of the Torah. All its typical institutions were committed to the care of the tribe of Levi, or to the priests, who were of that tribe; and it carries the seal of Divine origin. Chapter 18 defines private and domestic obligations which shall ensure purity in every relation of life. This did not only apply to the Jews, but to all nations of Canaan; and violations of these laws meant violation of nature itself. Intimate relationships within a nuclear family are forbidden. The nearest of kin is sister, mother, daughter; and the woman being born of the same flesh as the man is. The list includes other immediate relatives, including illegitimate sisters, half-sisters and step-sisters, step-mothers, grand-daughters, and women co-opted by a new family via marriage. Verses 12 to 14 include in this list of forbidden intimate relationships also aunts and uncles, both maternal and paternal, and maternal uncle's wife. Based on this principle, nieces are likewise excluded from those 'who shall not marry uncle or a nephew'. Daughters-in-law and sisters-in-law are reckoned truly daughters and sisters. Affinity and consanguinity are taken as equally important relationships, which shall not be violated by intercourse. It is declared to be 'horrid wickedness' to marry the daughter of a man's own step-daughter; much more, then, to marry the step-daughter herself.[139] Apart from detailed guidance on prohibited sexual relationships within a family clan, the script also defines approved practices relevant to preservation of population survival and long-term health. While the Book of Genesis describes formation and migration of tribes, the Book of Leviticus is a detailed description of survival and maintenance of viability of a tribe. The Book of Leviticus does not distinguish between 'mother' and 'mother-in-law' in terms of inappropriateness of an intimate relationship, no matter the latter would not be consanguineous, and uses both terms interchangeably as the term describes 'role' in family structure rather than blood relationship.

---

[139] Andrew Bonar. 1852. "Comments on the Book of Leviticus." James Nisbet and Company.

Ver. 6. None of you shall approach to any that is near of kin to him, to uncover their nakedness: I am the Lord.

Ver. 7, 8. The nakedness of thy father, or the nakedness of thy mother, shalt thou not uncover: she is thy mother; thou shalt not uncover her nakedness. The nakedness of thy father's wife shalt thou not uncover: it is thy father's nakedness.

Ver. 9-11. The nakedness of thy sister, the daughter of thy father, or (laughter of thy mother, whether she be born at home, or born abroad, even their nakedness thou shalt not uncover. The nakedness of thy son's daughter, or of thy daughter's daughter, even their nakedness thou shalt not uncover: for theirs is thine own nakedness. The nakedness of thy father's wife's daughter, begotten of thy father, (she is thy sister,) thou shalt not uncover her nakedness.

Ver. 12-14. Thou shalt not uncover the nakedness of thy father's sister: she is thy father's near kinswoman. Thou shalt not uncover the nakedness of thy mother's sister: for she is thy mother's near kinswoman. Thou shalt not uncover the nakedness of thy father's brother; thou shalt not approach to his wife: she is thine aunt.

Ver. 15, 16. Thou shalt not uncover the nakedness of thy daughter-in-law: she is thy son's wife; thou shalt not uncover her nakedness. Thou shalt not uncover the nakedness of thy brother's wife: it is thy brother's nakedness.

The Church did not appreciate the idea that humans were more than one species, and had anything to do with apes. Bruno (1591) and Vanini (1619) both put forward this idea, but the consequences for their daring theories were grave. Bruno was burned alive at the stake while Vanini's tongue was cut out before he was strangled at the stake and burned to ashes. With the rise of Christianity, the ape would turn into a 'figura diabolica', then to a sinner, and ultimately into a fool. Unlike Galen, Thomas Aquinas in his anatomical analysis found that there were no anatomical similarities between 'apes' and humans.[140]

---

[140] Brendan O'Flaherty, and Jill S Shapiro. 2002. "Apes, Essences, and Races: What Natural Scientists Believed about Human Variation, 1700-1900". Columbia University. Department of Economics.

While Carl Linneaus anchored his taxonomic description of four species of man in combination with connecting them with four temperament types according to the humoral theory of Ancient Greece without referring to the Bible, other biologist of that time, John Lyon Buffon in his History of Nature[141] directly referred to the Book of Genesis as the sole origin of all human races. Some references to the Bible and especially to the Hebrew Bible including the Book of Leviticus with regards to the need to maintain purity of a nation can be found in the Nazi ideology.

There is no consensus on what Hitler's belief system actually was. Some authors describe Hitler's faith as some sort of distorted form of Christianity, and compare the formation of new Aryan race to the new 'Chosen tribe' which is meant to replace the Jews who now for this very purpose have to be exterminated.

> 'This exceptionalism of the newly forming Aryan race, however, had a cultural foe since Jews claim Biblical chosenness, so
>
> a) the Bible had to be replaced in German consciousness by Germanic religion that became a cultic expression, and
>
> b) the 'other' chosen tribe had to be wiped out so Aryans could take their 'rightful' place in Human history as global leaders.'[142]

Other researchers concluded that either Nazism was an ideology which transformed morphed into a religion, or that the underlying faith was rooted in Celtic neo-paganism. The influences of late Nietzsche also had significant impact on Hitler's set of beliefs as later communicated through Mein Kampf. No matter what Hitler's religious and philosophical beliefs were, it is undisputed that its methods were rooted in social Darwinism taken to the extreme.

---

[141] John Lyon, Buffon, and Georges Louis LeClerq. 1976. "The Initial Discourse to Buffon's 'Histoire Naturelle.'" *Journal of the History of Biology* 9 (1): 133–81.

[142] Greg Chalik. "What Was the Relationship between Medical Profession and the Nazi State?" *Linked In; Group: Military History and Strategy; Discussion Thread: What Was the Relationship between Medical Profession and the Nazi State?*

THE POWER OF BLOOD AND PEDIGREE

The Levitican rules were here not only to prevent consanguineous intimate relationships which were likely to produce a defective offspring – which the priests were not concerned about as any malformed surviving persons would not be able to participate in reproduction in any case, and as individuals posed no threat to then society. The rules were mainly required to maintaining peace within family clans.

Religious prohibition of consanguineous marriages is by no means universal. In fact, cousin marriages, that are those where the couple shares at least one grandparent, account for more than 10% marriages globally; and in some cultures they are highly encouraged. Consanguineous marriages are particularly common in the Middle East, North Africa, and West Asia. In clinical genetics, a consanguineous marriage is defined by inbreeding coefficient equal or higher than 0.0156. This number represents a measure of the proportion of loci at which the offspring is expected to inherit identical genetic information from both parents. This definition includes unions between first and second cousins, as practiced among Arabs; and uncle-niece marriages as practiced in South India where inbreeding coefficient (F) reaches astonishing 0.125.[143]

Until early 20th century, blood unions between close relatives were also common in Western culture where marriages between closely related royals often resulted in hereditary disorders. In Medieval and Renaissance Europe, many if not most land acquisitions were realized through marriages between royals. Because of the preference of consanguineous marriages which were required to maintain elite status of the family, and to keep the property undivided, royal families were prone to accumulation of recessive alleles which could cause a disease, which would consequently follow the family throughout generations. One famous example is

---

[143]   Gonzalo Alvarez, Celsa Quinteiro, and Francisco C. Ceballos. 2011. *Inbreeding and Genetic Disorder, Advances in the Study of Genetic Disorders.* Edited by Dr. Kenji Ikehara. InTech.

the spread of hemophilia through the descendants of Britain's Queen Victoria to German and Russian imperial families. Queen Victoria's granddaughter Irene, daughter of her third daughter Alice, married her first cousin Prince Henry of Prussia, and gave birth to two hemophilic sons. Irene's sister Alix was also a carrier. Through marriage with Tsar Nicholas II she carried the disease into the Russian imperial family. The four healthy (non-carrier) daughters Olga, Tatiana, Marie, and Anastasia were not entitled to throne since they were women. Long awaited son Alexis, heir to the Russian throne, was born with hemophilia. All siblings were murdered during the Russian Bolshevik Revolution.[144]

Attempts to preserve purity of bloodline proved devastating to European kingdoms through the expression of rare diseases. It is not difficult to imagine that the concept of eugenics influenced concerns of British and Austrian imperial families over their own genetic health, especially in the face of military defeat at Sadowa in the case of Austria, and the need for military training of royal males which was incompatible with the diagnosis of hemophilia.

Obsession with purity of bloodline and pedigree manifested itself in all parts of English noble life, most importantly in adoration of purebred horses and dogs. The General Stud Book of English Thoroughbred was created in 1791 once the breed gene pool had been stabilized. All registered thoroughbreds have their pedigree traced back to the first foundation oriental Sires: Darley Arabian, Godolphin Barb, and Byerley Turk.[145]

Co-incidentally, the same year as the Brits founded their General Stud Book of English Thoroughbred as their contribution to humanity, the first ten amendments of the U.S. Constitution – The Bill of Rights – were ratified effective December 15, 1791. The 'Nobility clause' was already part of the U.S. Constitution since 1776. While maintaining noble pedigrees safe from malignant influences of inferior human types was subject to never ending discussions in Europe, American eugenics took different path

---

[144]   Yelena Aronova-Tiuntseva, and Clyde Herreid Freeman. "Hemophilia: 'The Royal Disease'. National Center for Case Study Teaching in Science". University at Buffalo, State University of New York.

[145]   TB Heritage. "Thoroughbred Heritage: Foundation Sires."

several decades later; and obsession with noble hereditary entitlements was certainly not its main driving force.

> 'No title of nobility shall be granted by the United States: and no person holding any office of profit or trust under them, shall, without the consent of the Congress, accept of any present, emolument, office, or title, of any kind whatever, from any king, prince, or foreign state.' (U.S. Constitution, Article I, Section 9, Clause 8)

Extreme example of equine inbreeding is the Kladruber horse, a heavy gala carriage baroque horse breed used by the Hapsburg imperial court for ceremonies. The breed is first mentioned in records from the era of Maxmillian II around 1552, and was elevated to a court stud in 1579 by Rudolf II with the financial support of the house of Fugger. There are two variants of the breed, gray – consisting of lines Generale, Generalissimus, Favory, and Rudolfo, and black – Sacramoso, Solo, Siglavy Pakra, and Romke. Its population is so small that a complex scheme of matching Sires and Dams has to be maintained to avoid inbreeding depression. The breed is considered a genetic rarity and it is a perfect example of purity of pedigree taken to the extreme.[146]

Arabian is another horse breed highly valued for its performance resulting from ruthless selection process and purity of pedigree. Arabian-type horses are all over the Middle East because Bedouins did not believe in gelding their colts and sold most of them, keeping only the most valuable ones. The genetic pool of 'pure' Arabian as it is known today was only reduced to five most valued maternal lines (Keheilan, Seglawi, Abeyan, Hamdani, and Hadban), together called 'Al-Khamsa', in 622 AD, following Mohammed's run from Mecca to Medina. The equestrian version of this story explains Mohammed's selection of the five primary maternal strains because they were the only five mares out of forty which turned their heads and came to their master when called by their name after they had finally reached water well following a long ride through the desert.

---

[146]   L Vostry, I Kracikova, B Hofmanova, V Czernekova, T Kott, and J Pribyl. 2011. "Intra-Line and Inter-Line Genetic Diversity in Sire Lines of the Old Kladruber Horse Based on Microsatellite Analysis of DNA." *Czech Journal of Animal Science* 56 (4): 163–75.

These five families of Arabian horses are still recognized as the only pure strains, and they mainly remain pure even within a strain since some tribes discourage even crossbreeding between strains.

This philosophy of extreme inbreeding in equine husbandry bears striking resemblance of preference of consanguinity in marriages throughout the Arab world. In early 7th century, Mohammed preached his monotheistic teachings to Meccans; but his opponents organized boycott against Muslim businesses and persecution against Muslims. After a foiled assassination plot Mohammed fled for Yathrib, a small oasis 200 miles north of Mecca; and hijira, as the event became known, was accepted as the beginning of Muslim era and Islamic calendar. The oasis was renamed to Madina-al-Nabi, the City of the Prophet, better known under its short name Medina. The 70 families that followed Mohammed to Medina became known as Mubajirun (those who made the hijira). Considering historical context of Mohammed's flight to Yathrib, the equestrian story about the purity of five Arabian strains is a reminiscence of the few faithful Mubajirun families.

It is hardly surprising that the methods used in the process of improvement of human race were taken directly from animal breeding. Just like farm animals not fit for reproduction were and still are routinely neutered and used either as work animals or as a for food; in Nazi Germany certain groups of people were banned from reproduction completely, some were sterilized, and some non-pedigree females from subjugated nations which expressed the right phenotype features were sent to 'breeding centers' where they were 'matched' with Aryan males. Exactly as domestic animals which were not selected as suitable for breeding get slaughtered and eaten, Jews and other not-good-enough races were used for slave labor and eventually disposed of in gas chambers.

The Eugenic Melting Pot (Europe in Turmoil)

One important driving force behind popularity of eugenics was gradual integration of Africans into overwhelmingly white society following abolition of slavery. Abolition of Slave Trade Act was passed through the British Parliament in 1807, but slavery only ended in 1834, and in reality it continued through apprenticeship schemes at least until 1838. Together with Portugal, Britain accounted for 70% of all Africans transported to the Americas including the Caribbean. Of the 3.1 million Africans transported by the British to their colonies in the period from 1640 to 1807, about 2.7 million survived the journey and reached their destination.[147] End of slave trade triggered profound changes in British economy and affected the whole structure of British Empire.

Apparently, economic destabilization following the Revolutionary War of Independence by enforcing abolition of slavery abroad was the motivation behind attempts to enforce this new rule on America, too. After the Declaration of Independence, Britain did not immediately give up ambitions to get its former colony back. In 1807, British frigate Leopard stopped USS Chesapeake to search it for Royal Navy deserters. James Barron's ship which had been refitted for further active service but not yet prepared for action quickly surrendered to the British. This was one of the incidents which eventually led to the War of 1812 between Britain and the United States.[148]

By 1812 westerners were convinced that driving the British out of Canada would solve their problems in the North, while war hawks of Georgia, Tennessee, and the Mississippi Territory used British-Spanish alliance against Napoleon as an excuse for invasion of Spanish-held Florida.[149] The British never recognized Napoleon as a legitimate ruler and considered his selling of vast Louisiana territory[150] to the USA[151] a fraud. This was used as justification of British plan to take New Orleans and continue along the Mississippi river to join forces coming down from Canada.

After the Battle of New Orleans (January 1815, the War of 1812) in

---

[147]   The National Archives. "British Transatlantic Slave Trade."

[148]   Naval Historical Center. "USS Chesapeake (1800-1813)."

[149]   Office of the Chief of Military History, United States Army. "American Military History, Army Historical Series: The War of 1812."

[150]   The Library of Congress. "American Memory: Louisiana: European Explorations and the Louisiana Purchase."

[151]   The Library of Congress. "Primary Documents in American History – Louisiana Purchase."

which General Jackson defeated Wellington's army, Britain had to give up hopes for restoration of its influence over America. They had other things to worry about, namely the Napoleon's army which was taking over the Continent (1796 – 1815), at least until June 1815, when Duke of Wellington and Gebhard von Blücher won over Napoleon at Waterloo.[152]

Eugenics was gaining popularity at time when European nobility felt threatened by political events unfolding around them and popular demand for higher involvement of the common man in governance. Scientific support of hereditary entitlements using biology and genetics benefited the nobility to justify their claim to power.

In historical context, Galton's 400 pages long tirade on indispensability of noble families for the well-being of mankind and progress of human race shrinks to a desperate attempt to prevent British Monarchy from falling apart. After a series of revolutions in 1848 and the establishment of French Second Republic, British Monarchy recognized popular demand for democracy on the Continent as a well-defined threat, and acted accordingly to protect the empire. The political landscape of Europe was profoundly changing.

Napoleonic wars led to adoption of rules for the treatment of wounded and sick in the battlefield, the Geneva Conventions of 1864. Henry Dunant, the founder of International Red Cross, in his book 'A Memory of Solferino' expressed a wish that each country should in peacetime set up a relief society which would aid the Army Medical Services in time of war and that the nations should ratify by convention a solemn principle which would give the necessary standing to such societies.[153]

In July 1866, one of the news headlines read: *'Prussian victory overthrows European order'*. It looked like if the old world was

---

[152]   Jeremy Black. 2008. *Great Military Leaders and Their Campaigns. Duke of Wellington, Pp 198-203.* Thames & Hudson.

[153]   Geneva International Committee of the Red Cross. 1952. "Geneva Convention for the Amelioration of the Condition of the Wounded and Sick in Armed Forces in the Field."

falling apart right in front of everyone's eyes. Möltke the Elder convinced King Wilhelm I of Prussia to attack the much larger Austrian army under Lajok von Benedek. The plan worked out due to Prussian army's superior firepower and organization. Möltke's Prussian army achieved an astonishing victory over the Austrian and Saxony army in the Battle of Sadowa (Battle of Königgrätz) in Eastern Bohemia. Three weeks later, the Austrian navy defeated the Italians in the Battle of Lissa[154] and Garibaldi's forces recaptured the City of Bezzecca in Northern Italy[155].

In the Battle of Sedan (1870), which followed another two victorious battles of Worth and Gravelotte, Möltke trapped the much smaller main French army and pounded it with his artillery. Napoleon III's decision to surrender not only ended his Second Empire, but also became known as the greatest French military disaster until the fall of France in 1940.[156]

The Seven Weeks' War resulted in passing political power in Germany from Austrian Hapsburg family to Prussian Hohenzollerns after four centuries of Hapsburg domination. Germany emerged as the strongest European power as a result of three successful wars fought by Prussia between the years 1864 and 1871, mainly due to the military genius of Möltke the Elder.

Eugenic ideas affected the way of thinking of leadership of European imperial armies during the Great War, either British, Austrian, Russian or German; as with increasing numbers of troops involved in the war the leadership displayed complete disregard for common man which was treated by officer ranks as 'inferior material'. Without widespread acceptance of scientific justification that value of certain groups of people is negligible, mass slaughter of entire generations of draftees would hardly be possible. The only place where extreme forms of social Darwinism took on even more malignant form than in Nazi Germany was Stalin's Soviet Union.

---

[154]   P Brewer. 2007. *The Chronicle of War. A Year-by-Year Account of Conflict from 1854 to the Present Day. P 62.* Carlton Books Ltd.

[155]   Jeremy Black. *Great Military Leaders and Their Campaigns: Giuseppe Garibaldi, pp 212-213.* Thames & Hudson. 2008.

[156]   Ibid. *Moltke the Elder, pp 214-217.*

Darwin and his Followers

19:19 Ye shall keep my statutes. Thou shalt not let thy cattle gender with a diverse kind: thou shalt not sow thy field with mingled seed: neither shall a garment mingled of linen and woolen come upon thee. (Leviticus, Chapter 19).

Eugenic movement was born in England from where it quickly spread to Germany as a result of efforts to describe nature including human race which was now perceived as part of the natural system, in contrast to the medieval concept of a distinct creature removed from its biological context.

Charles Darwin's Origin of Species was published in 1859 and his theory launched an avalanche of works which extended the rules he spelled out for animals to human race. Darwin's research was anchored in taxonomical works of Carl von Linne who identified about 7.700 known plants (published 1753) and 4.400 animals (1758) and gave them all a unique name which consisted of a genus and species, and created a classification system based on observable characteristics. Linne's 'Systema Naturae' (1735) also included people as a biological species. He described man as *Homo diurnus vagans cultura, loco,* and classified him as member of the Order Primates. His genus Homo recognized *Homo rufus, cholericus, rectus (Americanus)* as a distinct race of Native Americans; *Homo albus, sanguineus, torofus (Europeus)*; *Homo luridus, melancholicus, rigidus (Asiaticus)*; and *Homo niger, phlegmaticus, laxus (Afer)*; and *Homo monstrosus.* The classification reflected then generally accepted humoral theory of four temperaments as known from Ancient Greece.

Other theories, such as that these different types are in fact a distinct genus and not mere species were soon disregarded because of typical characteristics of inter-genus hybrids which are typically infertile while this is not the case among humans who form inter-racial unions as they feel like and as their cultural environment permits. Between 1749 and 1788, French philosopher John Lyon Buffon published three volumes of his History of Nature, of which one was dedicated to 'Man'. Like most French philosophers of that time, Buffon believed that all humans belonged to one original stock which could be traced back to the tribes described in the

Book of Genesis; however, some of them degenerated over time due to exposure to extreme environments. Buffon explained differences between people by the influences of climate, soil, terrain, and air, and concluded that hot climate led to idleness and passivity.[157]

Ten years after the publication of Darwin's Origin of Species (1859) and two decades after the French Revolution of 1848, Darwin's cousin Francis Galton published his 'Hereditary Genius'. More research and publications on the same topic soon followed. In 1874, Galton published 'English Men of Science'[158], series of works on anthropometry, psychometry, and fingerprinting[159] (1879 to 1895), and most notably 'Essays on Eugenics' (1909), 'Natural inheritance' (1889), 'Race Improvement - The possible improvement of the human breed under the existing conditions of law and settlement' (1901-2), 'Our national physique-prospects of the British race-are we degenerating?' (1903), 'Eugenics – Its definition, scope and aims' (1904), 'Studies in eugenics' (1905), 'A eugenics investigation: index to achievements of near kinsfolk of some of the Fellows of the Royal Society' (1905), 'Eugenics: I. Restrictions in marriage' and 'II. Studies in national eugenics' (1906), 'Probability, the Foundation of Eugenics' (1907), 'Local associations for promoting eugenics' (1908), 'Address on eugenics' (1908), 'Deterioration of the British Race' (1909), 'Eugenic qualities of primary importance' (1910), and eventually interview 'Eugenics and the Jew' (1910).

While Francis Galton was the most prolific author on eugenics, he was not the only one. Eugenics, anthropometrics, and related disciplines were becoming mainstream science freely discussed in international conferences. In 1868, Ernst Haeckel published his 'Natural History of Creation' (1868), but it took three decades for another wave of similar works to emerge. Towards the end

---

[157] Elizabeth Rechniewski. 2004. "The Significance of Aesthetic Prejudice in French Enlightenment Commentaries on Human Variety." *Literature and Aesthetics* 14 (2): 67–83.

[158] Francis Galton. 1873. *English Men of Science: Their Nature and Nurture.* Histoire des Sciences et des Savants depuis deux Siecles. Par Alphonse de Candolle. Corr. Inst. Acad. Sc. de Paris, &c. Geneve.

[159] Francis Galton. *Finger Print Directories.* Macmillan. 1895.

of the 19th century, Alfred Ploetz published 'The Excellence of our Race and the Protection of the Weak' (1895), and started a magazine 'Archive for Racial and Social Biology' (1904); and Wilhelm Schallmayer's Heredity and Selection in Peoples' Generations' (1903) came to light.

Galton's Hereditary Genius (1869)

The idea of eugenics came from amateur British scientist Sir Francis Galton who extensively utilized research of his uncle Charles Darwin. In his first book *'Hereditary Genius*'[160] which was published in 1869 Galton argued that 'good' and accomplished families were more likely to produce intelligent and talented offspring. Here he presented a 'case for nobility'.[161] In 1889, Galton published his *'Natural inheritance*'[162], and his most influential book *'Essays in eugenics*'[163] followed in 1909.

All these works were first published in Britain in apparent reaction to the French Revolution of 1848 which was considered a grave threat to the British Empire. Conservative Victorians did not believe in the idea that governments could be dissolved by threats and violence; and did not think that constitutions should be extracted by force from below. British Empire reacted to the Chartists challenge in 1848 rather violently and the parliamentary leaders emphasized the need for protection of private property. Great Britain remained neutral and insisted on the preservation of law and order[164].

The book Hereditary Genius is over 400 pages long and starts with a very distinguished pedigree. Galton extended research in hereditary traits in plants to humans and drew conclusions

---

[160]   Francis Galton. *Hereditary Genius*. Macmillian & Co, London 1869, and New York 1892.

[161]   Eugenics: "America's Darkest Days."

[162]   Francis Galton. *Natural Inheritance*. Macmillan & Co, London. 1889.

[163]   Francis Galton. *Essays in Eugenics. Eugenics Education Society.* London: Macmillan & Co, London. 1909.

[164]   University of Ohio. "Great Britain And The Revolutions of 1848." *Encyclopedia of 1848 Revolutions.*

which he believed should be adopted as an official policy. His main concern was whether persons who belong to the 'highest classes' with regards to success in honorable professions contribute their fair share in reproduction, and that higher fertility of 'less valuable stock' does not lead to degeneration of human race:

> *"The striking results of an evil inheritance have already forced themselves so far on the popular mind, that indignation is freely expressed, without any marks of disapproval from others, at the yearly output by unfit parents of weakly children who are constitutionally incapable of growing up into serviceable citizens, and who are a serious encumbrance to the nation."* *(Hereditary Genius, p xx)*

Galton's theory was later used in some African colonies where certain indigenous people were given power over other tribes based on perceived racial and class superiority. The most illustrative example of such practice was German-Belgian colony Rwanda in Central Africa where Tutsi minority was granted priority access to positions within state administration and allowed to rule this way over Hutu majority which was effectively locked away from access to education and state administration[165]. This scheme did not work out very well because it produced lot of anguish which eventually resulted in violence and genocide.[166]

> *"The varieties of Negroes, Bantus, Arab half-breeds, and others who now inhabit Africa are very numerous, and they differ much from one another in their natural qualities. Some of them must be more suitable than others to thrive under that form of moderate civilization which is likely to be introduced into Africa by Europeans, who will enforce justice and order, excite a desire among the natives for comforts and luxuries, and make steady industry, almost a condition of living at all."* *(Hereditary Genius, p xxvi)*

Galton classified men by their reputation and natural gifts, and wrote separate chapters on some selected professions such as the

---

[165] Troy Riemer. "How Colonialism Affected the Rwandan Genocide."

[166] Romeo Dallaire. *Shake Hands with the Devil. The Failure of Humanity in Rwanda*. Da Capo Press. 2004.

Judges, statesmen, commanders, and literary men, men of science, poets, musicians, painters, oarsmen, and wrestlers; and in the concluding part he compared the results with different races and assessed influences that affect the natural abilities of nations. Little attention is paid to other nations such as Italians and Jews, Americans and Germans but the reasons for their omission is desire to avoid glaring errors. *'It is a little less so with respect to France, where the Revolution and the guillotine made sad havoc among the progeny of her abler races' (p 4).* From remarks like this it is obvious that Galton did not appreciate the French Revolution at all and made his stance clear in this work in which he appreciated the value and heritage of distinguished English families.

> *'To conclude, the range of mental power between—I will not say the highest Caucasian and the lowest savage—but between the greatest and least of English intellects, is enormous. There is a continuity of natural ability reaching from one knows not what height, and descending to one can hardly say what depth.'* *(Hereditary Genius, p 26)*

On several occasions Galton compared hereditary traits in humans to those in domestic animals, including breeding and selection process. He was mainly interested in talents, dispositions, character, and fertility, and took great care to count numbers of descendants and relatives of distinguished families. Some of the tables of pedigrees of English statesmen, judges, and commanders produced by Galton do not provide any supporting argument for his statements at all because they are based on false logical reasoning. Galton neglected to mention that Judges, statesmen, men with literary and scientific accomplishments, and military commanders were rarely selected from the ranks of common men, and that distinguished families are more numerous in certain professions as a direct result of selection bias and rather than their inherited superiority. By describing distinguished families in selected professions and their kinship as evidence of better quality of human stock Galton presented a perfect circular argument. Hereditary Genius was the first Galton's work and it was so significant mainly because of the historical context at time of publication.

THE LOW END

The Jukes (1874)

Twelve years after the end of American Civil War, RL Dugdale published a long study 'The Jukes, A record and study of the relations of crime, pauperism, disease, and heredity', about a clan of criminals descending from Mother of all criminals, for the purpose of Dugdale's study codenamed Ada Juke. This study was later used in many works as a basis for many measures taken against hereditary criminals, harlots, and the chronically poor. In 1874, the author of this study visited thirteen county jails of the State New York and examined pedigrees of some of these prisoners. Blood relationships were labeled by family name 'Juke' whilst relations by marriage and cohabitation were marked as 'X'.

Illegitimate branch of Ada Juke produced 49 adults of Juke bloodline and 32 adults of those associated with the Jukes by marriage or cohabitation. Of these 81 people, 15 Jukes and 5 'X' became convicted criminals who served almost 80 years of prison sentence in total. Positive statistics does not explain the causes and can be mistaken with correlations and coincidences. According to Dugdale, criminals show larger percentage of illiteracy than the average community, therefore illiteracy is the cause of crime. Dugdale paid attention to the Theory of probabilities and statistics, and was careful not to draw causal relationships from correlations he observed.

In the study of pathology of social disorders, many of them caused by organic disease of body or mind, he considered critical assessment essential whilst statistics only a part of the exploration. Fornification, extra-marital sex, was the backbone of their habits, flanked on one side by chronic poverty (pauperism) and on the other by crime. Secondary features are prostitution, which produces illegitimate children (bastards). Child neglect and ill-education then results in exhaustion and intemperance and imbalanced minds, disease, and eventually extinction.

The study is dedicated to family line called the Jukes, which counted 709 persons related either by blood or by marriage and cohabitation, and produced extraordinary number of criminals. At the same time, he examined the ratio between marriageable women and harlots in the Jukes family and the 'X' line, and numbers of legitimate and illegitimate children. Dugdale argues that harlotry may become a hereditary characteristic; and that this can be stopped by environmental factors and early marriage. Prostitution in women is analogous to pauperism and crime in men. Illegitimacy is not considered a risk factor, as illegitimate children placed in favorable conditions may succeed in life better than legitimate children in the same conditions; it is the environment of neglect which is mischievous.

The last section is dedicated to the amount of charity received by the Jukes over lifetime, both from private and public funds. Pauperism is an indication of weakness of some kind, and can be either hereditary or induced. Whilst accidents of life are not hereditary, induced pauperism can become hereditary through establishments of habits. Younger children are more likely to become the inmates of poorhouse through misconduct or misfortune of their parents.

Further down in the text Dugdale presented statistics of crime depending on various demographic characteristics including age, gender, and legitimacy, history of child neglect, education, and poverty. This classification with regards to crime has not changed substantially to the present day. It is difficult to understand how this study could have been used as the main argument for eugenics, and for sterilization of 'habitual criminals'. The text does not suggest that the relationship between number of criminals within a family and phenotype is causal and biologically determined. In fact the author carefully distinguishes between hereditary and environmental factors and states that one has to be careful not to confuse co-incidence with causality. Dugdale stressed the importance of environmental factors which are frequently associated with social pathologies, such as child neglect as a consequence of illegitimacy, ill-health as a consequence of inherited conditions and poverty rather than simple indolence, or premature death as a consequence of pauperism and criminal career. Of the 709 family members included in this study, most spent considerable part of their lives either in prison or in a poorhouse.

Significant part of the study focuses on term 'neurosis', in an apparent effort to find a link between violence and epileptic fits, a phenomenon which is explained as a 'convulsion of ideas' rather than convulsion of muscles. In conclusion of his study, Dugdale listed typical classes of criminals and raises the question how shall their numbers be decreased? As per experience, three years of separate imprisonment have better effect than ten years of congregate custody because of lack of recognition by co-prisoners after release and obliteration of sense of self-respect by longer detention. Where individual cure cannot be accomplished, extinction of criminal race has to be organized. Whilst in the past this was usually achieved by hanging, now the preferred route is long-term isolation of the criminal and placing of children in benign environment which benefits their normal development.[167]

The Quest for Causes of Crime

Dugdale was not the only scholar who was trying to analyze causes of criminal behavior from demographic characteristics of convicts. These efforts were typical for 19th century criminology in the USA as means of prevention of violent crime and elimination of pauperism as behavioral and lifestyle characteristics. As per the Pearson Education, explanations of criminal behavior fall into eight general categories: classical, biological, psychobiological, psychological, sociological, social process, conflict, and emergent. According to classical and neoclassical theories, which were the most relevant before the emergence of eugenic theories, crime is caused by individual exercise of free will and the most important determinants of human behavior are pain and pleasure; and as per Beccaria (1784), the punishment should fit crime and should not be excessive.

Before the Civil War, the dominant theory of crime deterrence was based on hypothesis of 'free will' based risk assessment when pursuing any illegal activities. Punishment was there to outweigh the rewards.[168] In this sense, criminal career was a result of rational

---

[167] RL Dugdale. 1891. *The Jukes. A Study in Crime, Pauperism, Disease, and Heredity, Also Further Studies of Criminals.* G.P. Putnam's Sons, The Knickerbocker Press.

[168] Jeremy Bentham. *Philosophy of Utilitarianism (1748–1832).*

choice. But the eugenics movement in medicine affected criminology the same way; and biological theory of crime started gaining more popularity. One can only speculate how much the liberation of slaves after the Civil War contributed to the emergence of theories of biological determination of criminal and other pathological behavior. Basic assumptions of this biological theory of criminal characteristics were that human behavior is determined either constitutionally or genetically and these traits are passed from one generation to next.[169]

Whilst Dugdale in his study on clan of poor white farmers codenamed 'The Jukes' was very careful to define 'hereditary' conditions as those which are passed down either through genetics or through environment, and non-hereditary factors, many other observers and propagators of his work failed to observe this clear distinction and falsely assumed that 'hereditary' means 'inherited' in biological sense of this term. It might seem that this criminological study, which is cited in nearly all important materials on eugenics, was seriously misinterpreted over time. A tale of genetic immorality was born out of this distortion. Scientists, doctors, judges, politicians, and clergy advocated 'eugenic marriage laws' to prevent families like 'The Jukes' from threatening everyone else's well-being and polluting the gene pool.[170]

The era of eugenics in the U.S. did not last very long. Some laws, including those on compulsory sterilizations were still passed and enforced. By the Great Depression, geneticists largely disavowed poverty as genetic condition. In 1939, John Steinbeck confronted the idea of hereditary poverty caused by degeneration in his novel The Grapes of Wrath, in which he followed the fate of the family of white farmers impoverished by rapid industrialization of agriculture in the Great Plains. He did not think that the Joads, as the family was called, were inferior to corporations which were buying out their traditions and livelihood for a pittance after a

169   F Schmalleger, Pearson Education, Inc,. 2009. "Criminal Justice Today" Pearson Prentice Hall, New Jersey.

170   D Vergano. 2012. "Myth of the Jukes Offers Cautionary Genetics Tale." *USA Today*, July 2.

series of bad harvests caused by extreme drought.[171]

Robert Shilkret in his review of book "*Mental retardation in America: A historical reader*" compared the Jukes and the Kallikaks[172] to Steinbeck's Lennie Small and Faulkner's Snopes family, as a confrontation of inter-generational societal problems within families which were at that time taken as a proof of inherited degeneracy.[173]

Many theories gained popularity at those times and contributed to wide acceptance of eugenics within scientific and medical communities and the general public. Phrenology, a science about human skull and relation of certain features to human behavior[174], was later used by the Nazis for much more malignant purpose. For example, Cesare Lombroso (1835-1910) argued that criminals share certain anatomic defects that are specific for them; and their numbers can be reduced in future generations by preventing children from being born into their families. Those who become criminals only through contact with people with undesired characteristics would have less opportunity to become vicious if there were lower numbers of habitual criminals.

The author concluded that vasectomy is safe for the patient, does not represent a punishment for the criminal because it does not result in deformity, neither it endangers his life, nor interferes with his enjoyment of life. The operation was performed under local anesthesia consisting of combination of morphine and cocaine in sterilized water. As per the author, this treatment would do away with hereditary criminals from the father's side and aside from being sterile the criminal would retain his normal condition. This method would protect the community at large without

---

[171] John Steinbeck. 1939. *The Grapes of Wrath*.

[172] HH Goddard. *The Kallikak Family: A Study in the Heredity of Feeble-Mindedness*. Toronto, Ontario: Classics in the History of Psychology. Christopher D. Green, York University.

[173] R Shilkret. 2004. "Mental Retardation in America: A Historical Reader. The History of Disability." Edited by Steven Noll and James W. Trent, Jr. *Bulletin of the History of Medicine. New York: New York University Press* 79 (2): 354–55.

[174] Franz Joseph Gall. "Phrenology."

harming the criminal. The same could reasonably be suggested for inebriates, imbeciles, perverts, and paupers.[175]

In the late 19th century, American public came to conclusion that the growing population of prisoners and the mentally ill is resulting in racial suicide, and the eugenic movement gained in popularity. The socially inadequate included people with certain mental illnesses such as mania or schizophrenia; dependents such as the deaf, blind, and physically deformed; the degenerates, e.g. sadists and drug abusers; the delinquents, such as the wayward and criminals; people who were mentally deficient like the morons and idiots; and those infected with tuberculosis, syphilis, and lepers.[176] This way of thinking resurfaced later during the Tuskegee experiment in which natural course of untreated syphilis was observed in black males. Belief that there is nothing wrong with this approach was likely caused by lack of entitlement to healthcare in combination with effort to keep certain groups of people out of reproduction.

Positivist school of criminology, which was invented by Lombroso, borrowed the term atavism from Charles Darwin. According to Lombroso's teachings, born criminals express certain primitive features such as e.g. long arms, large lips, crooked nose, large amount of body hair, and certain shape of ear lobe. This theory was in 1913 disproved by Goring and Pearson who felt that Lombroso's research methods were inadequate; and to prove the point they compared 3,000 English convicts to army officers just to find no significant differences between the two groups. This research was published in The New York Times in 1919 by Walter Littlefield.[177]

In 1939, Ernest Hooten, firm believer in Lombroso's concept of a born criminal identifiable by physical characteristics, thought that

---

[175] AJ Ochsner. 1899. "Surgical Treatment of Habitual Criminals." *JAMA* 32: 867–68.

[176] MJ Drake, IW Mills, and D Cranston. "The Eugenics Movement. Quoted and from 'The Chequered History of Vasectomy.'" *British Journal of Urology.*

[177] Walter Littlefield. 1919. "Criminal Is a Defective, but Not a Type; Conclusions from Biometrical Study of 3,000 British Convicts Discredit Lombroso's Theory and Minimize the Influence of Environment." *The New York Times*, December 21.

there was a general agreement concerning the physical attributes of races but no consensus concerning the link between biological features of a person and his personality or propensity for deviance. In 1927, Hooton began his massive project in which he intended to prove correctness of Lombroso's theories that deviant behavior is a result of 'low-grade mentality'.[178]

The same year, the Supreme Court overturned the decision on unconstitutionality of eugenic sterilizations, and eugenics began slowly but surely taking root in Germany, reaching completely new horizons. None of these measures would be imaginable without wide acceptance of eugenics as a concept by the general public.

---

[178]   KB Melear. 1998. "The Criminological Theory of Earnest A. Hooton; Theory in Criminology and Criminal Justice" Florida State University.

AMERICAN EUGENICS

Eugenic movement first came to America with Galton's works in the 1870's, but only spread toward the end of 19th century due to the 1892 International Congress on Demographics in London where Galton presented his research and his books. Many American scientists attended the congress. One of the consequences of increasing interest in eugenics in the U.S. was the establishment of institutions such as Davenport's Eugenics Record Office in 1910. Unsurprisingly, the strongest popular support for eugenics in the U.S. occurred with intense industrialization and culmination of the Great Depression in the 1920s and 1930's. In the period between the years 1900 and 1909, when the public debate on eugenics became most intense, the most fiercely discussed topics of the day were science as a way of creating a better race of human beings, optimization of quality of offspring through better selection of mate, and suppression of less desired races and social groups in favor of well-educated and thriving white middle class.

Eugenics became the mantra of the day just like political correctness of these days; and was aggressively promoted in American newspapers as the best possible cure for all societal problems related to marriage and quality of population. Big part of the public debate related to definition of the right human stock, especially in parts of the country which were racially more homogenous. Whilst Africans and other people of color were the prime targets of the eugenics debate, the most vilified for their danger to society were poor whites because they were not so easily distinguishable from the 'good white families'; and threatened to pollute the gene pool with their hereditary inclination to pauperism, crime, and harlotry. Some eugenicists were not scared to label them as outcasts.

The first law on inappropriateness of interracial marriage was enacted in Maryland 1664. The clause even included enslavement of them and their children as punishment for white women who dared to intermarry with Negro slaves.

"For as much as diverse freeborn English women forgetful of their free condition and to the disgrace of our Nation do intermarry with Negro slaves by which also diverse suits may arise touching the [children] of such women and a great damage doth befall the Masters of such Negroes for prevention whereof for deterring such freeborn women from such shameful matches, Be it further enacted by the authority advice and consent aforesaid that whatsoever freeborn woman shall intermarry with any slave from and after the last day of this present Assembly shall serve the master of such slave during the life of her husband, and that the [children] of such freeborn women so married shall be slaves as their fathers were. And be it further enacted that all the [children] of English or other freeborn women that have already married Negroes shall serve the masters of their parents till they be thirty years of age and no longer."

In 1691, interracial marriages were banned as abominable in Virginia, and the law threatened those who marry people of color and produce spurious children with '*Negroes, Mulattos, and Indians*' with removal from dominion. Fine of fifteen pounds sterling was to be paid to the Church wardens of the parish, the child shall be enslaved, and the woman disposed of for five years. By 1900, twenty six states implemented anti-miscegenation laws. In 1871, Rep. Andrew King (D-MO) proposed an amendment to the U.S. Constitution which would ban all marriage between whites and people of color throughout the United States.

In November 1881, Tony Pace and Mary J Cox were indicted and imprisoned according to the Section 4184 and 4189 of the Code of Alabama. They challenged the conviction all the way to the U.S. Supreme Court. In the case Pace vs. Alabama (1883)[179] the plaintiff claims that 'discrimination is made against the colored person in the punishment designated, which conflicts with the clause of the fourteenth amendment prohibiting a state from denying to any person within its jurisdiction the equal protection of the laws.' The precedent would stand for another 81 years, until slow change of the tide in the McLaughlin vs. Florida (1964)[180] and eventual

---

[179] *Pace v. State of Alabama.* 1883. U.S. Supreme Court.

[180] *McLaughlin vs. Florida.* 1964. U.S. Supreme Court.

complete overturn in the Loving vs. Virginia (1967)[181] case. In the words of George Tucker Harrison (1900), *'The negro occupies, according to anthropologists, the lowest position on the evolutionary scale.'* Harrison's argument was mainly based on examination of skulls which supposedly provided clues determining the person's intelligence and character traits. The most remarkable difference identified in the brains of Africans imported to America was an overdevelopment in the areas governing emotions and underdevelopment in the cognitive areas.

The most significant works in American eugenics include study by Daniel Kevles 'In the Name of Eugenics: Genetics and the Uses of Human Heredity' and numerous monographs and articles by Garland E. Allen. Assistant Secretary of Agriculture W.M. Hays was not scared to extend the experience with farming and animal breeding to human race, and emphasized the potential of eugenics:

> *'The subject of investigating the heredity of man is comparatively much more difficult than in the case of plants and animals. But it is so important that science and religion should join in an investigation at once conservative, careful, and possibly constructive.'*

Dr. Eugene Davenport of the University of Illinois as the most aggressive propagator of eugenics proposed that:

> *'all the 'culls' or 'scalawags' of the human race should be taken before the courts, scientifically investigated, and if found unworthy, colonized and permitted to die off.'*

---

[181]   *Loving v. Virginia.* 1967. U.S. Supreme Court.

Perhaps the most influential anthropologist of those days was physician of Czechoslovak (then Austrian-Hungarian Empire) descent Aleš Hrdlička whose main contribution to the field of eugenics was foundation of The *American Journal of Physical Anthropology (1918),* and the American Association of Physical Anthropologists (1929). Already in 1903 he began to organize the division of physical anthropology at the U.S. National Museum, which later became the Smithsonian Institution, where he acquired one of the largest collections of human bones in the world.

In the early 20th century eugenicists like Garret P Serviss, Daniel Kevles, or Eugene Davenport managed to get corporate support for their discipline. They established several institutions based mainly on the East Coast. The movement's most charismatic leaders eventually pushed through eugenic-based legislation such as the sterilization laws at state-level. Dr. H.W. Anderson, president of the California State Eugenics Association, understood eugenics' mission as 'labor to produce a better race of human beings'. In early 1900's, very few protagonists of eugenics openly called for marriage restrictions based on solely legislation principles. One of the major opponents of legislative measures for marriage based on eugenic principles was Alexander Graham Bell who believed that

> *'American society wished to produce the finest progeny, and that this desire alone would shape marriage and breeding practices for the nation'*

and that

> *'mere dissemination of that knowledge would of itself tend to promote desirable and prevent undesirable unions of the sexes.'*

Probably the most radical proponent of elimination of certain groups from reproduction was criminal anthropologist Lyndston who openly promoted sterilization of the *'criminal, epileptic, drunken, and the insane'* because of the danger to society they represented.[182]

---

[182]   Celeste Sharpe. "A Better Race of Human Beings: Eugenics in the American Media 1900-1909". University of Calgary. 2011.

Sterilization laws in America

In 1899, Dr Ochsner of Augustana and St Mary's hospital in Chicago published an article 'Surgical treatment of habitual criminals'[183] in which he advocates vasectomy as a humane method of ensuring that criminals as a class do not reproduce. He described two case reports of successful resection of vasa deferentia in patients who suffered from prostate problems. Ochsner's argument was that it has been demonstrated without a doubt that large proportion of all criminals, perverts, and degenerates come from parents who are affected in a similar way, and suggested vasectomy as a humane alternative to castration. Whilst vasectomy prevents people with undesired behavioral and physical characteristics from having children and protects society, the procedure does not result in any disability and does not affect the person's quality of life including his ability to enjoy sex. The author was not overly worried about females because they were likely to contract venereal disease early in life and become infertile this way. For females, ligation and resection of Fallopian tubes was suggested as an alternative to naturally occurring venereal diseases. When it eventually came to implementation of sterilization laws in the USA, females were sterilized almost as often as males.

The first sterilization laws in the United States were passed in 1907 in Indiana. The most prominent advocate of vasectomies of 'defectives' to prevent transmission of degenerate traits was Harry Clay Sharp who at meetings of the American Medical Association convinced many fellow physicians to lobby for laws allowing the involuntary sterilization of 'sex offenders, habitual criminals, epileptics, the feeble-minded, and hereditary defectives' because of the burden they imposed on society by production of social dependants.

The surgeon of possibly the highest professional standing to speak in favour of eugenic sterilization was Dr William Belfield, Professor

---

[183]   AJ Ochsner. 1899. "Surgical Treatment of Habitual Criminals." *JAMA* 32: 867–68.

of Surgery at Rush Medical College, who listed factors encouraging crime as:

> 'The farcical maladministration of our medieval criminal laws, the notorious partnership between criminals and many public officials and the maudlin sentiment which has infinite compassion for the prisoner but none for those of us who keep out of jail'.

Washington was the second state to pass a sterilization law in 1909. The law referred to habitual criminals and those convicted of rape or carnal abuse of female persons under the age of ten. The statute was challenged in 1912 by Peter Feilen who was in September 1911 convicted of rape of a female under the age of ten but the law upheld. In January 1921, another bill was passed which aimed to sterilize every patient in Washington mental hospitals and the state institutions for the feeble-minded. This bill was invalidated in 1942. According to Joanne Woiak the legislation is now used very rarely as a punitive measure; but in historical context the operation was offered as a method of birth control.[184] The total number of sterilized under this clause was 685, which was about 7 persons per 100,000 inhabitants.[185]

Washington Revised Code RCW 9.92.100: Prevention of procreation.

> Whenever any person shall be adjudged guilty of carnal abuse of a female person under the age of ten years, or of rape, or shall be adjudged to be an habitual criminal, the court may, in addition to such other punishment or confinement as may be imposed, direct an operation to be performed upon such person, for the prevention of procreation.
> [1909 c 249 § 35; RRS § 2287.][186]

---

[184] Joanne Woiak. *History of Eugenics in WA State.*

[185] Lutz Kaelber. 2012. "Washington: Eugenics: Compulsory Sterilization in 50 American States. Available At:" presented at the Social Science History Association.

[186] *Washington Revised Code: 1909 c 249 § 35; RRS § 2287, Prevention of Procreation. 1909 c 249 § 35; RRS § 2287.*

By far the largest number of sterilizations was performed in the state of California where until 1964, in total 20,108 people, mostly those mentally ill or 'deficient', were sterilized according to eugenic sterilization laws starting 1909. This number accounted for about one third of all 63,678 eugenic sterilizations in the United States in 26 states where these laws were enacted with Virginia (7,162), North Carolina (6,297), Michigan (3,786), Georgia (3,284) and Kansas (3,032) leading the way.

Harry H Laughlin, the author of five-hundred-page long monograph *'Eugenical sterilization in the United States'* became the most important proponent of policy change with regards to putting these ideas into practice. In the 1920's there was no federal statute regulating sterilizations of the 'unfit' but there were already fifteen states which did pass such laws but five of them had their laws either vetoed by governor or revoked by popular referendum.[187] For example the Oregon State Board of Eugenics ordered to carry out 2,341 sterilizations in total according to Oregon Eugenics law which was signed into law in 1917. The Oregon eugenics law continued to be used until the 1960s until it was eventually repealed in 1983.[188]

Eugenic policies manifested themselves also in immigration legislation. In response to the growing influx of immigrants from Southern and Eastern Europe as a result of changes after the World War I, the U.S. Congress passed in 1921 the Quota Act, and in 1924, the Immigration Act. The Act limited immigration of people of inferior races, especially those from Southern and Eastern Europe.[189]

---

[187] Alex Wellerstein. 2011. "States of Eugenics: Institutions and Practices of Compulsory Sterilization." In *California Reframing Rights: Bioconstitutionalism in the Genetic Age*, edited by Sheila Jasanoff, 29–58. Cambridge, Mass.: MIT Press.

[188] Lutz Kaelber. "Oregon: Eugenics: Compulsory Sterilization in 50 American States".

[189] *U.S. Immigration Act of 1924*. 1924.

Number of eugenic sterilizations carried out in the United States

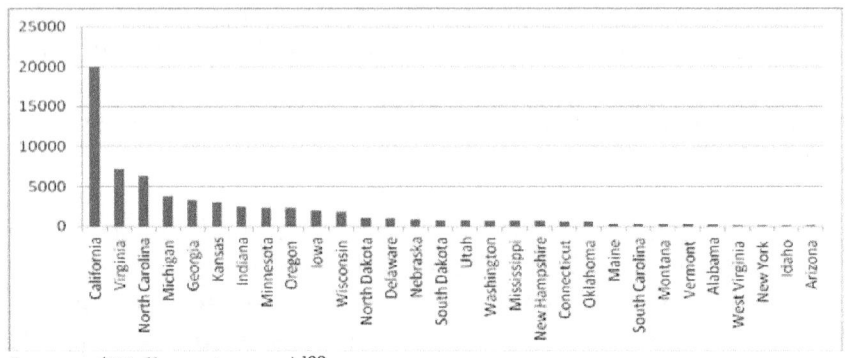

Source: (Wellerstein, 2011)[190]

Immigration quota as per the 1924 U.S. Immigration Bill

Country	Quota	Country	Quota	Country	Quota
Germany	51227	Poland	5982	Africa (other than Egypt)	1100
Great Britain and Northern Ireland	34007	Italy	3845	Armenia	124
Irish Free State (Ireland)	28567	Czechoslovakia	3073	Australia	121
Sweden	9561	Russia	2248	Palestine	100
Norway	6453	Yugoslavia	671	Syria	100
France	3954	Romania	603	Turkey	100
Denmark	2789	Portugal	503	Egypt	100
Switzerland	2081	Hungary	473	New Zealand & Pacific Islands	100
Netherlands	1648	Lithuania	344	All others	1900
Austria	785	Latvia	142		
Belgium	512	Spain	131		
Finland	471	Estonia	124		
Free City of Danzig	228	Albania	100		
Iceland	100	Bulgaria	100		
Luxembourg	100	Greece	100		
Total (Number)	142483	Total (Number)	18439	Total (Number)	3745
Total (%)	86.5	Total (%)	11.2	Total (%)	2.3
(Total Annual immigrant quota: 164,667)					

Source: Statistical Abstract of the United States (Washington, D.C. 1929)

---

[190]   Alex Wellerstein. 2011. "States of Eugenics: Institutions and Practices of Compulsory Sterilization." In *California Reframing Rights: Bioconstitutionalism in the Genetic Age*, edited by Sheila Jasanoff, 29–58. Cambridge, Mass.: MIT Press.

In 1924, the 18-year-old 'feeble-minded white woman' Carrie Buck, the daughter of a feeble-minded mother, both committed to the State Colony in the state of Virginia, was ordered to undergo salpingectomy for the purpose of becoming sterile. The Circuit Court argued that if the woman was discharged from the institution as sterile, she would pose no risk to society through undesired procreation. In 1927 the U.S. Supreme Court affirmed this decision as Constitutional:

> 'In view of the general declarations of the legislature ... they justify the result. We have seen more than once that the public welfare may call upon the best citizens for their lives. It would be strange if it could not call upon those who already sap the strength of the State for these lesser sacrifices, often not felt to be such by those concerned, in order to prevent our being swamped with incompetence.
>
> It is better for all the world if, instead of waiting to execute degenerate offspring for crime or to let them starve for their imbecility, society can prevent those who are manifestly unfit from continuing their kind. The principle that sustains compulsory vaccination is broad enough to cover cutting the Fallopian tubes. [Jacobson v. Massachusetts]. Three generations of imbeciles are enough.
>
> But, it is said, however it might be if this reasoning were applied generally, it fails when it is confined to the small number who are in the institutions named and is not applied to the multitudes outside. It is the usual last resort of constitutional arguments to point out shortcomings of this sort. But the answer is that the law does all that is needed when it does all that it can, indicates a policy, applies it to all within the lines, and seeks to bring within the lines all similarly situated so far and so fast as its means allow.
>
> Of course, so far as the operations enable those who otherwise must be kept confined to be returned to the world, and thus open the asylum to others, the equality aimed at will be more nearly reached.' [Buck vs. Bell, 1927][191]

---

[191] U.S. Supreme Court. 1927. *Buck v. Bell*. U.S. Supreme Court.

In 1974, Virginia repealed its 1924 law allowing state-enforced sterilization without overturning the 1927 U.S. Supreme Court decision. By the year 1930, 50,000 Americans were sterilized by enforcing the eugenic laws. With the ascent of Nazi Germany the popularity of the movement waned; and in 1939 the Eugenic records office was finally closed.

In 1942, in another landmark case, Skinner vs. Oklahoma 1942, U.S. Court reverted this ruling as discriminatory. Justice William Douglas noted that

> 'Sterilization of habitual offenders in no way guarantees that new offenders will not be born. Furthermore, there is no guarantee that habitual offenders would spawn offenders themselves.'

Chief Justice Harlan Stone concurred in the judgment, but rested his decision on due process grounds, arguing that the invasion of personal liberty is too great.[192] However, sterilization of the mentally ill continued until 1975. In the 1970's, the movement would take on a new form. This time, the prime targets of reproductive infringements were Native American women. About a quarter of this population became forcibly sterilized as late as in 1976. These measures were accepted by the public due to the eugenic theories which argued that Indians are a separate species.

Not in all conquered territories the colonizers attempted to force eugenics and racial segregation. According to Patrick Wolfe, there was a difference in approach to eugenics depending on interest of the colonizers. If they were more interested in labor, they would keep the subjugated peoples separate, and discourage miscegenation in order to maintain supply of slaves who were distinct from the ruling class. But should they be more interested in land, the perceived gain would be different, and intermarriage between the conquerors and the conquered would be encouraged to assimilate the indigenous population in the white stock.

Moreover, the culture of the household was defined by that of the husband rather than the wife. For this reason, intermarriage between white women and black or Native American males would be discouraged while the other way round miscegenation did not

---

[192]   *Skinner v. Oklahoma Ex Rel. Williamson. 1942.*

represent a problem.[193]

The eugenic movement gained public approval in the context of the Great Depression which made white families seriously struggle; and that's what made the societal problems much more apparent. Unemployment and economic insecurity caused intense anxiety and made many couples to put off starting their families until much later. This is apparent from the demographic development during the Great Depression when fertility rates dropped by 20% in the period from 1928 to 1935. World War Two brought some recovery because of the improved economic prospects and industrial power base America provided to its European Allies, and later for its own participation in the war. But full recovery only occurred after the war, when the birth rate increased to 113.4 per 100,000 women in childbearing age (15 to 44).

Fertility rates in the U.S. during the Great Depression

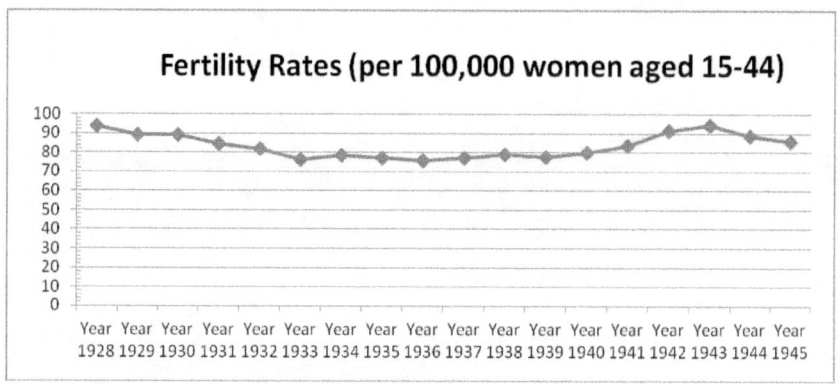

Source: Shmoop - The Great Depression Statistics

The power of the Constitution

The question whether what happened in Nazi Germany could ever happen in America is not difficult to answer: it did not happen. Eugenics was greatly popular and widely accepted first by the scientific community and eventually by the general public, but even when the movement was at its peak, not all the states passed

---

[193] D Forbes. 2011. "Compulsory Sterilization of Native Americans and Racist Motivations Behind Public Policies". SOC297 Independent Study, Prof. Lutz Kaelber, Dept. of Sociology, University of Vermont.

sterilization laws to stop their undesirables from reproducing. In fact half of the states did not implement eugenic laws at all. Full third of more than 60,000 eugenic sterilizations in the United States was performed in the Golden State. In 1927 the practice of eugenic sterilizations of the feeble minded was challenged as unconstitutional in the Buck vs. Bell[194] case but at that time the law was affirmed. With the onset of Nazism in Germany the popularity of eugenics began rapidly declining.

The end of era of American eugenics did not come with the defeat of Nazi Germany or Supreme Court rulings. It only came when Americans reconciled their relationship with their intellectually disadvantaged fellow citizens and embraced a character like Forrest Gump as integral part of society, not as a liability, but part of its success.

---

[194]   U.S. Supreme Court. 1927. *Buck v. Bell.* U.S. Supreme Court.

THE ULTIMATE EUGENICISTS

The Aryan Race

Among the many influences on Hitler's Mein Kampf, Friedrich Nietzsche was the most fundamental one. Nietzsche, the author of 'The Genealogy of Morals', considered himself anti-democratic, anti-Christian, anti-Judaism, and anti-socialist. Nietzsche's sister Elisabeth Förster-Nietzsche who became the most important protagonist of his works and who created what is called the 'legend of Nietzsche' also reconciled the work with that of Richard Wagner. To finance maintenance of her brother's archive Elisabeth introduced his prophetic and radical philosophy to her preferred National Socialist party and even made friends with Herr Hitler. Nietzsche's theories found very fertile ground in Hitler through Elisabeth Förster-Nietzsche. Hitler was captivated by the rhetoric of condemnation of the slave race, adoration of the new Aryan superman, and the proposed Darwinistic solution. Mein Kampf was philosophically anchored in Nietzsche's theories. His blond beast, synonymous with the 'complete man' or a 'whole man' is a symbol of greatness and untamed human potential unrestrained by values; a human who never experienced resentment because that was only reserved for the weak for revenge against the strong. Slaves were detestable men for both Nietzsche and Hitler. Nietzsche associated the 'magnificent blond brute' with the Roman, Arabic, Germanic, and Japanese nobility. Just like Nietzsche's 'blond beast' (*The Genealogy of Morals*), German 'Teuton beast' was destined to reach mankind's full potential. In the defense of horrors of extermination of the weak, Nietzsche argued that it is better to be afraid of the impulsive and strong than 'the dwarfed, stunted, and envenomed'.[195]

By the 1870's extermination of inferior races had already received significant support among Darwinist writers as 'inevitable result of clash between cultures'. In the 1880's scientific racism in Germany radicalized even further due to Ludwig Gumplowitz

---

[195] Michael Kalish. "Friedrich Nietzsche's Influence on Hitler's Mein Kampf". UCSB. 2004.

who developed his Darwinism-inspired sociological theory of group conflict, which he published in 1884 under the title 'Racial Struggle'. Friedrich Ratzel's 'Lebensraum' (living space) presented as a theory of colonization and warfare was later used to justify German imperial expansion as a genuine 'need'. Population expansion justified territorial expansion. Around 1900 the eugenicist rhetoric was becoming increasingly inflammatory, and also disseminated widely through Europe and especially Germany. A leading eugenicist, Professor Max von Gruber, openly advocated imperialist expansion. Others, like Willibald Hentschel and Heinrich Driesmans, were openly promoting extermination of inferior races.

In 1896 Alfred Ploetz published a book in which he introduced concept of racial hygiene into German thought. Although eugenics only reached its peak in Germany with World War Two, its ideas helped justify the previous global conflict also. Eugenicists worked hard to support assertion of Germany in Europe as the dominant power; and if some of them such as i.e. Haeckel later presented themselves as pacifists it was for the wrong reasons. In their opinion, the main problem of modern warfare was not the mass slaughter it inflicted but that the 'wrong people died'. Because most of the casualties of war were those who were fit and strong, the war was seen as counter-selective. Immediately before the start of World War One, Eugene Fischer published a book about mixed-blood people of Southwest Africa, arguing that they shall be offered minimal protection as 'a race inferior to ourselves'. Once World War One broke out, eugenicists' opposition to war dissolved completely.[196] World War One then brought rationing which led to widespread deaths from starvation of psychiatric patients in German hospitals since they were low priority. Eugenicist ideas that they should be in fact left to die as low value humans also contributed to their discarding as dispensable.

In the early interwar years Hoche and Binding came up with publication 'Permission to destroy life unworthy of life' which rationalized medical killing and argued that right to life has to be

---

[196]   Richard Weikart. 2003. "Progress through Racial Extermination: Social Darwinism, Eugenics, and Pacifism in Germany, 1860-1918." *German Studies Review* 6.

earned, not assumed. Negative eugenics slowly took root in German mind. Medical killing was rationalized as removal of diseased part of society and understood as 'therapeutic'. The idea to eliminate the crippled, the insane, and the criminal to free up resources required by the worthy ones was prophetic. When Hitler's Mein Kampf was published in 1925 and 1926, it was not perceived as controversial reading at all. In fact it fit well among all other eugenicist works of that time and only became enormously popular even before Hitler's rise to power due to philosophical context and vision for Germany which resonated not only with the Party members but to great extent with the nation as whole.

In recent years, Hitler and Mein Kampf gained popularity in India where it does not have the stigma of mass murder. Main Kampf became a best-seller and a must read for many business school applicants. European history gets limited time in Indian schools but in the context it gets is Hitler's contribution to Indian independence. Without Nazi Germany weakening Great Britain the colonizers would have never left on their own. With India's affinity to strong military leaders, Hitler is perceived as a hero.[197]

Homo Sovieticus

In the Soviet Union eugenics and social Darwinism took on a completely different form, in a way complementary to that adopted by the Nazis. Homo Sovieticus, the most valued product of Soviet human breeding, was the product of Bolshevik revolution once all pernicious elements such as intellectuals, bourgeoisie, independent farmers, and members of competing political parties were safely disposed of either in labor camps or by other means. The methods were essentially the same, only the selection criteria and killing methods were different.

In practical terms, selection of targets of public outrage followed familiar pattern known from Nazi Germany. The first victims of Bolshevik purges were those who were economically successful. Stalin rejected the idea of eugenics in favor of Lysenkoism. In 1936, American geneticist Hermann J. Miller wrote a letter to Stalin in

---

[197]   David Shaftel. 2012. "Hitler Has a Following in India." *Bloomberg Business Week*, December 6.

which he advocated creation of a eugenic program in the USSR. Miller spent the period between December 1934 and September 1937 in Moscow, where he held a position of Senior Geneticist at the Institute of Genetics of the U.S.S.R. Academy of Sciences on the eve of the great purges. After receiving the letter, Stalin had Miller's book '*Out of Night*' translated in Russian. As a great believer in environmental egalitarianism, Stalin in 1937 ordered an attack on all genetics, protecting the neo-Lamarckism and Lysenkoism. Except for population improvements achievable only in a socialist system compare to bourgeois society Miller was also concerned about the potential of artificial insemination of women whose chances of getting married were minimal due to the absence of males in their area caused by war, not mentioning the purges.[198]

While state-imposed breeding programs for own citizens may be over for now, some societies still practice elaborate schemes of marital matching which give very little freedom to choose one's life partner. These programs are less motivated by population health and quality of an offspring rather than preservation of a family clan in some traditional form.

---

[198] John Glad. 2003. "Hermann J. Muller's 1936 Letter to Stalin." *The Mankind Quarterly* 43 (3): 305-19.

V. LEGACY

Twentieth century, with its spread of ideologies which denied existence of God and Supreme justice, introduced change of thinking within the medical profession. It does not mean previous conflicts and epidemics were less deadly or less devastating. It only means that they did not challenge the existence of God within the medical profession. This changed with the series of doomsday cults which followed abolition of serfdom in Russia, and culminated in Bolshevik revolution of 1917 toward the end of World War One, and with the spread of national and international socialism which transformed ideology into religion. All-powerful new human races, Homo Aryan and Homo Sovieticus, were there to take over. Medical profession played crucial role in ascension of these malignant regimes, both Communist and Nazi, and in creation of these new human species, which would be better and cleaner and closer to a specific ideal than previous naturally occurring types, just like livestock quality which improves with better breeding. Some doctors took up the role of not priests but Gods. Not a healthy move for a man; and certainly not a healthy move for a society. The journey from The Hague and Geneva Conventions to the Nuremberg laws and the Helsinki Accords, the Belmont report and the CIOMS guidelines was long and ragged, and littered with bodies of people killed in violation of these newly adopted standards. These rules did not emerge out of nowhere and were always proposed, discussed, commented, and adopted in the context of conflicts and civil rights movements which were taking place at that time.

SCIENTIST'S MIND

The use of domestic prisoners for drug testing was considered perfectly acceptable by the public until the 1970's when series of scandals and consequent acceptance of the Belmont Report stopped this practice as unethical. Post-war development then gave way to formulation of international standards in medical experimentation and medical care. Medical experiments conducted by the Nazi Germany and by Imperial Japan on whole groups of low value people shook the entire world. This historical experience is still part of collective memory in most cultures due to the fact that these atrocities were well documented and extensively taught at schools at all levels from elementary to universities. Nuremberg military tribunal with war criminals included investigation of crimes against humanity committed in concentration camps by Nazi doctors in the name of science in a situation of supposedly non-existent standards for conducting of clinical experiments. The argument of non-existence of regulations in clinical research before the World War Two is fundamentally flawed since the standards did indeed exist on German territory. They were disregarded by the scientific community itself with the ascent of Nazi Germany, by shifting attention from an individual to the society, and by embracing eugenics as an ideology which justified killing of 'unworthy life'. The most important conclusion of the Nuremberg trial was that some principles of humanity are given and do not have to be formally stated in written legal form to be formally prosecuted as crimes against humanity in a military tribunal settings. The Nuremberg trial sparked interest in ethical standards in clinical research, and adoption of the Universal Declaration of Human Rights. But non-consensual clinical research did not end with the World War Two. It was not eliminated by making representatives of various countries to sign and ratify standards of civilized behavior. The practice of the use of prisoners, prisoners of war and civilian population of local undesirables for medical experiments continued both at time of war and at time of peace.

The Nuremberg Medical Cases

In preparation of the trial, Nazi defendants were given an IQ test. All of them scored higher than average. The graphic footage displayed in the courtroom during the trial was essential to comprehend the full extent of the scale of the atrocities. Despite overwhelming evidence, the Nazi leaders continued to claim that they were unaware of the atrocities and felt little personal responsibility because they only followed orders. 'Butcher of Poland' Hans Frank put it best:

"Don't let anyone tell you they had no idea! Everybody sensed that there was something horribly wrong with this system, even if we didn't know all the details. They didn't want to know!"[99]

The trial with major war criminals defined crimes against humanity as murder and ill-treatment of prisoners of war and civilians, pillage of public and private property, slave labor policy, and persecution of the Jews.[200]

Medical experiments on prisoners of war and civilians were tried in the Nuremberg Medical Trial 1, 2, and 4. Case 1, the USA vs. Karl Brandt, was a trial against 23 doctors and administrators accused of organizing and participating in war crimes and crimes against humanity in the form of medical experiments and medical procedures inflicted on prisoners of war and civilians. Experiments with the effects of high-altitude flying on humans were conducted at Dachau camp using freezing temperatures and low-pressure chambers built for this purpose. Seawater was tested on prisoners if it can be made drinkable. More than a thousand Dachau prisoners were used for the research of malaria and development of a vaccine. In Sachsenhausen, Natzweiler, and other camps, experiments with mustard gas and epidemic jaundice were performed on prisoners in order to find treatment to benefit German armed forces. Experiments with infectious diseases such as typhus, cholera, small pox, and others, were conducted in concentration camps

---

[99] A Walker. *Nazi War Trials*. Pocket Essentials. 2006.

[200] *Nazi Conspiracy and Aggression: Opinion and Judgment. Office of United States Chief of Counsel for Prosecution of Axis Criminality.* 1949. Washington, DC: U.S. Government Printing Office.

Buchenwald and Natzweiler. Poisoned food and phenol was tested in Buchenwald, as well as treatments of phosphorus burns. Poisoned bullets were tried in Sachsenhausen. In Ravensbrueck, efficacy of sulfanilamide was tested on infected wounds of prisoners, as well as experiments with muscle, bone, and nerve regeneration, and bone transplant experiments. In Auschwitz and Ravensbrueck, experiments with large scale sterilization were performed using X-rays, drugs, and surgery, in order to exterminate enemy population. At Auschwitz, 112 Jews were killed for the sole purpose of getting their skeleton for collection. Experiments with phlegmon were conducted in Auschwitz and Dachau. Polygal was tested on prisoners for its efficacy for the treatment of wounds. Tuberculosis became a reason for killing in occupied Poland based on public health concerns. Secret killings of the aged, insane, incurably ill, and deformed took place all over Germany. In Case 2, USA vs. Erhard Milch, the charges included medical experiments with high altitude and freezing on German nationals and citizens of other countries. Case 4, USA vs. Oswald Pohl, specified charges as medical experiments, sterilization, euthanasia, and extermination of Jews.[201]

Extermination of entire population segments was carefully planned long in advance and the plan was systematically executed. If the war lasted longer, there would not be many Jews left. Needless to say, the Jews were not the only group affected by systematic exploitation and killing. 'Inferior' races and nations, 'undesirables' of all kinds, and those 'unfit for life in Reich' were affected the same way. The Nuremberg military tribunals could by no means hold accountable every single person who willingly participated in this mass atrocity.

Consent of whole society was essential for murders on this scale. The Tribunal pointed out direct responsibility of businesses which directly invested corporate money in research on subjects who did not consented to it in order to promote their own business interests. For vast majority of Germans, extermination of entire groups of people became psychologically and morally justified, especially in situation when elimination of competitors resulted

---

[201] Harvard Law School. "Nuremberg Trials Project." *Harvard Law School Library: Nuremberg Trials Project.*

in monetary rewards, career opportunities, or access to abandoned property.

Medical experiments in which nobody sought the consent of subjects to testing occurred relatively independently in several different places in the world. The main impulse for this came from the scientific community itself. It was the demand for new knowledge, recognition for innovative research, and demand for scientific characteristics of medical experiment which required 'material' for testing, as well as economic need. Important condition of such conduct was dehumanization of some people who were either not entitled to any care or were perceived as liability for the society as whole.

For emerging authoritarian governments, economic boom resulting from medical research was a great boost which helped financing the rise of Nazism. At the same time, the added value of 'improvement of overall health and quality of the population' was immediately understood as a great opportunity to decrease costs of care and dispose of dissent and opposition. Fear of becoming 'fodder' quickly split the society in two camps: executioners and victims.

How the ends rationalize the means

General public did not object. Benefits of such conduct were explained as public health matter. A 100 human guinea-pigs would save countless lives if their 'sacrifice' was used for example for the development of vaccine against a deadly disease. This argument earned support due to the Spanish Flu pandemic which broke out in the end of the First World War and easily killed more people than the war had. The total number of people killed in combat during the war reached approximately 8.5 million on all sides. The total number of casualties including the wounded, prisoners of war, and missing in action is estimated around 37.5 million[202]. Compared to this, Spanish Flu killed 20 to 40 million people in just one year[203]. Statistically, it is not difficult to justify experiments on a minority to protect majority against a disease like flu.

---

[202]   Department of Justice. "WWI Casualty and Death Tables. U.S. Casualties in Major Wars."

[203]   Molly Billings. "The Influenza Pandemic of 1918."

The most important condition of general approval of mass murder and medical experiments which result in physical or mental harm, is overwhelming sense of impunity of those engaged in these activities. Positive feedback and peer pressure from within the scientific community draws into the pathological vicious circle even those who would otherwise stay away.

Dehumanization of certain segments of population helps to soothe ones conscience in the beginning, whilst later the most important motivation becomes satisfaction rooted in sense of superhuman power, latent sadism, or shared feeling of guilt. Limited means of defense available to victims and survivors further facilitated the sense of impunity. General population is unlikely to object out of fear of becoming victims.

Physicians as the driving force of Nazi policies

Professor Seidelman in his paper 'Nuremberg lamentation: for the forgotten victims of medical science'[204] analyzed the relationship between medical profession and the state, and the ways this profession entered the slippery slope of large scale killing of segments of the population, and how it became one of the pillars of dictatorial regime. The main paradigm of medical practice in Nazi Germany was to improve overall health of the nation' by positive selection and removal of those who do not fit the desired standard. The interests of an individual who is disabled, gravely ill, or has undesired physical or mental characteristics, are in direct contradiction of 'society', which only wishes to have people who are healthy, look good, and do not require extensive and expensive medical care.

In section 'State misuse of professional power', Prof Seidelman defines broader questions and challenges for medical profession arising from the Nuremberg trial. Apart from the previously mentioned client relationship between state and medical profession which excludes patient from decision-making and reduces him to passive recipient of care, there are other points which explain the problem more precisely: the physicians were loyal to the state

---

[204]   William E Seidelman. 1996. "Nuremberg Lamentation: The Forgotten Victims of Medical Science." *BMJ*, 313.

for political and socioeconomic reasons; and secondly, the physicians had the right and power to decide whether the person would be treated or not based on his value for society. The role of physician-teacher and physician-scientist became a vehicle for profound political and social change.[205]

Hartmut M Hanauska-Abel in his paper 'Not a slippery slope or sudden subversion: German medicine and National Socialism in 1933' discusses the two most widely accepted concepts of downfall of German medicine, known as 'slippery slope' and 'sudden subversion'. Based on evaluation of documents published in German journals in 1933, Hanauska-Abel states that the German medical community completely lost the moral ground already in 1933, and even in some respects outpaced the new government, what means it hardly was barely victim of circumstances but one of the initiators of the political and social change.[206] In 1932, director of the Kaiser-Wilhelm Institute of Psychiatry Munich Ernst Rudin became president of International Eugenic Congress. He was the main author of the idea of sterilization of people with mental illnesses and genetic disorders, and positive population measures to keep the nation healthy and energetic.

The T4 euthanasia program was turned into a highly profitable industry. The 'safe disposal' of over 70.000 futile or terminally ill patients was then calculated in monetary terms of food which did not have to be provided to those who had no capacity to pay.

Acceptance of the concept of extermination of 'subhuman' races was aggressively spread and widely accepted in the German medical community. Hitler was appointed a Chancellor on January 30, 1933. Barely two months later, on March 21, 1933, Dr A Stauder, democratically elected president of two largest German medical associations met his fellow Nationalist Socialists for intimate talks regarding 'the political revolution', and telegraphed Hitler that the principal medical organizations gladly place themselves at the

---

[205] Ibid

[206] Hartmut M Hanauske-Abel. "Not a Slippery Slope or Sudden Subversion: German Medicine and National Socialism in 1933." *Medicine & Global Survival.* 1996.

service of this great patriotic task. The service was by no means selfless but very well paid. In 1933, after Hitler came in power, the medical and lawyer community aggressively expelled non-Aryan professionals and the salaries began to rise steeply[207]. The main driving force in medical profession was greed.

The chosen few

In Nazi Germany, the profession as a whole shifted its loyalty from service provided to an individual patient to service provided to the state already under the Bismarck's regime. Hitler's coup was the critical condition for further shift of focus of medicine toward interests of the state because it gave doctors guarantees of impunity. Medical professionals in Nazi Germany became a superhuman caste with unique social status directly responsible to the National Socialist Party.

In Communist countries, becoming a doctor was the highest point on the Communist social ladder a commoner could achieve. This definition of a commoner excluded substantial numbers of citizenry on the grounds of 'politically reliability'. Physicians in the Soviet Bloc had immense authority and their skills and intentions were never questioned. This social exclusiveness exempted medical profession from any public scrutiny. Any misconduct, medical errors, lack of judgment or knowledge, or corruption was always dismissed or blamed on money and resources but never on lack of skills, knowledge, effort, or will. This God-like status created sense of superhuman powers and total impunity for any shortcomings within the profession.

The same phenomenon can be observed in Indian society due to the historically ingrained caste system where those who practiced medical profession belonged to the high classes. This perception of own exceptional status if unchallenged can result in gross malpractice and misconduct due to missing feedback mechanism. In 2011, an article was published in The Independent on testing of pharmaceuticals on people belonging to low classes

---

[207] Ibid

of Indian society, and on survivors of the Bhopal gas disaster.[208] The main concerns raised in this article were that no investigation into deaths relating to the trials were conducted; patients who were unaware of the fact that they were enrolled in a clinical trial and therefore could not provide consent with the experiment; existence of a serious conflict of interest within the hospital ethics committee where the doctors acted as trial facilitators what made it nearly impossible for the patients to say no; and inadequate consideration of safety hazards in trial protocols. Since 2009, more than 1,500 clinical trials involving more than 150,000 subjects were started in India. The series of articles in The Independent blamed corporate greed and western neocolonialism, and lack of oversight. However, without national governments turning blind eye to widespread exploitation of their own population by their own native doctors, this widespread abuse would never be possible.

---

[208]   N Lakhani. 2011. "From Tragedy to Travesty: Drugs Tested on Survivors of Bhopal." *The Independent*, November 15.

BIBLIOGRAPHY

A Walker. 2006. *Nazi War Trials*. Pocket Essentials.

AH Maehle. 2012. "God's Ethicist: Albert Moll and His Medical Ethics in Theory and Practice." In *Medical History*, 56 (2):217–36. Published by Cambridge University Press.

AJ Ochsner. 1899. "Surgical Treatment of Habitual Criminals." *JAMA* 32: 867–68.

Alex Wellerstein. 2011. "States of Eugenics: Institutions and Practices of Compulsory Sterilization." In *California Reframing Rights: Bioconstitutionalism in the Genetic Age*, edited by Sheila Jasanoff, 29–58. Cambridge, Mass.: MIT Press.

Amanda Schaffer. 2006. "A President Felled by an Assassin and 1880's Medical Care." *The New York Times*, July 25.

American Medical Association. 1847. "Code of Medical Ethics of the American Medical Association". American Medical Association Press.

American Medical Association. "Ethics Timeline: 1847 to 1940."

Andrew Bonar. 1852. "Comments on the Book of Leviticus." James Nisbet and Company.

Bednar, Marek, Vera Frankova, Jiri Schindler, Andrej Soucek, and Jiri Vavra. 1996. *Lekarska Mikrobiologie*. Marvil.

Bokser, Rabbi Ben Zion. 2013. "Moses Maimonides." *Encyclopedia Britannica*.

Boris Volodarsky. 2009. *The KGB's Poison Factory from Lenin to Litvinenko, pp32-48*. Frontline Books. Zenith Press.

Bowdoin College. 2014. "Bowdoin: The Mongol Invasions of Japan 1274 – 1281." *Bowdoin: Asian Studies*.

Brendan O'Flaherty, and Jill S Shapiro. 2002. "Apes, Essences, and Races: What Natural Scientists Believed about Human Variation, 1700-1900". Columbia University. Department of Economics.

Brett McKay, and Kate McKay. "The Bushido Code: The Eight Virtues of the Samurai." 2008.

Broughton, Methew J. "Catapulted Death: Can a Flying Corpse Distribute the Plague?" *Insects, Disease, and History*.

C Mackenzie. "German Firm Which Invented Birth Defect Drug Thalidomide Apologizes for the First Time in 50 Years - but British Charity Demands Compensation." *Daily Mail*.

C Timmermann. 2001. "A Model for the New Physician: Hippocrates in Interwar Germany." In *Reinventing Hippocrates*, 302–24. Centre for the History of Science, Technology and Medicine, University of Manchester.

C. H. W. Johns. "The Avalon Project. Source: Babylonian and Assyrian Laws, Contracts and Letters, (1904), One of a Series Called the Library of Ancient Inscriptions, from a Facsimile Produced by The Legal Classics Library, Division of Gryphon Editions, New York in 1987."

Celeste Sharpe. "A Better Race of Human Beings: Eugenics in the American Media 1900-1909". University of Calgary. 2011.

Chamberlain, Neal R. "Lymphoreticular and Hematopoetic Infections: Plague." 2010.

Chapin, Laura. "Mitt Romney and the GOP's War on Birth Control." *US News*, February 6, 2012.

Cohn, SK, and LT Weaver. 2006. "The Black Death and AIDS: CCR5-_32 in Genetics and History." *QJM* 99 (8): 497–503.

Cragin, Kim, and Sara A Daly. 2004. "The Dynamic Terrorist Threat - An Assessment of Group Motivations and Capabilities in a Changing World." RAND Prepared for the United States Air Force.

D Forbes. 2011. "Compulsory Sterilization of Native Americans and Racist Motivations Behind Public Policies". SOC297 Independent Study, Prof. Lutz Kaelber, Dept. of Sociology, University of Vermont.

D Guyatt. "Deep Black Lies. Unit 731."

D Vergano. 2012. "Myth of the Jukes Offers Cautionary Genetics Tale." *USA Today*, July 2.

Daniel Fu-Chang Tsai, and Ding-Shinn Chen. 2003. "An Oath for Bioscientists." *Journal of Biomedical Science* 10: 569–76.

Daqing Yang. 2006. "Documentary Evidence and Studies of Japanese War Crimes: An Interim Assessment." In *Researching Japanese War Crimes Records: Introductory Essays*, 21–56. National Archives and Records Administration for the Nazi War Crimes and Japanese Imperial Government Records Interagency Working Group.

David Shaftel. "Hitler Has a Following in India." *Bloomberg Business Week*. 2012.

Debroy, B. "A New Hippocratic Oath. The Indian Express", July, 2007.

Department of Defense. "Overview of the Pearl Harbor Attack, December 7, 1941." *Naval History and Heritage Command*.

Department of Justice. "WWI Casualty and Death Tables. U.S. Casualties in Major Wars."

Des Ormeaux, AL. 2007. "The Black Death and Its Effect on Fourteen and Fifteen Century Art." Graduate Faculty of the Louisiana State University and Agricultural and Mechanical College.

Durham University. 2014. "Moll Project. Sexuology, Medical Ethics, and Occultism."

E Drea, G Bradsher, R Hanyok, J Lide, M Petersen, and D Yang. 2006. "Nazi War Crimes and Japanese Imperial Government Records Interagency Working Group." In *Researching Japanese War Crimes Records Introductory Essays.*, 79–110. Japanese War Crimes Records at the National Archives: Research Starting Points. Washington D.C.

"Edward III (1327-1377)." 2014. *The Official Website of the British Monarchy*.

Elizabeth Rechniewski. 2004. "The Significance of Aesthetic Prejudice in French Enlightenment Commentaries on Human Variety." *Literature and Aesthetics* 14 (2): 67–83.

Ellen Rice. 2007. "Dr. Frances Kelsey: Turning the Thalidomide Tragedy into Food and Drug Administration Reform."

F Drobniewski. 1993. "Why Did Nazi Doctors Break Their 'Hippocratic' Oaths?" *Journal of the Royal Society of Medicine* 86: 541–43.

F Schmalleger, Pearson Education, Inc,. 2009. "Criminal Justice Today" Pearson Prentice Hall, New Jersey.

FDA. "Kefauver-Harris Amendments Revolutionized Drug Development."

Francis Galton. *English Men of Science: Their Nature and Nurture*. Histoire des Sciences et des Savants depuis deux Siecles. Par Alphonse de Candolle. Corr. Inst. Acad. Sc. de Paris, &c. Geneve. 1873.

Francis Galton. *Natural Inheritance*. Macmillan & Co, London. 1889.

Francis Galton. *Finger Print Directories*. Macmillan. 1895.

Francis Galton. 1909. *Essays in Eugenics. Eugenics Education Society*. London: Macmillan & Co, London.

———. "Eugenics: America's Darkest Days."

Francis Galton. *Hereditary Genius*. Macmillian & Co, London 1869, and New York 1892.

Franz Joseph Gall. "Phrenology."

Geneva International Committee of the Red Cross. 1952. "Geneva Convention for the Amelioration of the Condition of the Wounded and Sick in Armed Forces in the Field."

"German History in Documents and Images: Volume 7. Nazi Germany, 1933-1945; Law for the Restoration of the Professional Civil Service (April 7, 1933)." 1933.

Gimbel, LM. 2012. "Bawdy Badges and the Black Death: Late Medieval Apotropaic Devices against the Spread of the Plague". A Thesis submitted to the Faculty of the College of Arts and Sciences of the University of Louisville.

Gonzalo Alvarez, Celsa Quinteiro, and Francisco C. Ceballos. 2011. *Inbreeding and Genetic Disorder, Advances in the Study of Genetic Disorders*. Edited by Dr. Kenji Ikehara. InTech.

Greg Chalik. "What Was the Relationship between Medical Profession and the Nazi State?" *Linked In; Group: Military History and Strategy; Discussion Thread: What Was the Relationship between Medical Profession and the Nazi State?*

H Wing. 1969. "Louis Lasagna, Life, Death, and the Doctor." *Valparaiso University Law Review* 3 (2, Art 11): 318–20.

Hammurabi, and King LW (translator). "The Code of Hammurabi."

Hartmut M Hanauske-Abel. "Not a Slippery Slope or Sudden Subversion: German Medicine and National Socialism in 1933." *Medicine & Global Survival* 3. 1996

Harvard Law School. "Nuremberg Trials Project." *Harvard Law School Library: Nuremberg Trials Project.*

Harvey, AE. 1982. *Jesus and the Constraints of History*. Westminster John Knox Press.

HH Goddard. *The Kallikak Family: A Study in the Heredity of Feeble-Mindedness*. Toronto, Ontario: Classics in the History of Psychology. Christopher D. Green, York University.

Hippocrates, and Ludwig Edelstein (Translation, interpretation). 1943. "From The Hippocratic Oath". Baltimore: Johns Hopkins Press.

Hulkover R. 2010. "The History of the Hippocratic Oath: Outdated, Inauthentic, and Yet Still Relevant." *The Einstein Journal of Biology and Medicine*, 41–44.

Ibeji, Mike. 2011. "Black Death." *BBC History.*

Islamic Philosophy Online, Inc. 2014. "The Muslim Philosophy."

James McNaughton. 2006. *Nisei Linguists: Japanese Americans in the Military Intelligence Service during World War II. Map 15, Pp 388-389.* Department of the Army, Washington D.C.

Jeremy Bentham. *Philosophy of Utilitarianism (1748–1832).*

Jeremy Black. 2008a. *Great Military Leaders and Their Campaigns. Duke of Wellington, Pp 198-203.* Thames & Hudson.

———. 2008b. *Great Military Leaders and Their Campaigns: Admiral Nimitz, Successful Commander of American Naval Forces against Japan, Pp 274-9.* London: Thames & Hudson.

JH Tanne. 2003. "Louis Lasagna." *BMJ* 327 (7414): 565.

JM Kleeberg. 2003. "From Strict Liability to Workers' Compensation: The Prussian Railroad Law, the German Liability Act, and the Introduction of Bismarck's Accident Insurance in Germany, 1838-1884." *International Law and Politics* 36: 53–132.

Joanne Woiak. *History of Eugenics in WA State.*

Joel Price. 2014. "Writing a Code of Ethics Writing a Code of Ethics." *Scholars Portfolio Education Specialist.* Accessed May 10.

John Glad. 2003. "Hermann J. Muller's 1936 Letter to Stalin." *The Mankind Quarterly* 43 (3): 305–19.

John Lyon, Buffon, and Georges Louis LeClerq. 1976. "The Initial Discourse to Buffon's 'Histoire Naturelle.'" *Journal of the History of Biology* 9 (1): 133–81.

John Steinbeck. 1939. *The Grapes of Wrath.*

JR Silver. 2003. "The Decline of German Medicine, 1933-45." *J R Coll Physicians Edinb* 33: 54–66.

Jun Hongo. 2007. "Vivisectionist Recalls His Day of Reckoning. Doctor Put Conscience on Hold until War Atrocity Confession Time Came. October 24, 2007." *The Japan Times Online*, October 27.

K Baker. "The Doctors Who Killed a President." *The New York Times*. 2011.

KB Melear. 1998. "The Criminological Theory of Earnest A. Hooton; Theory in Criminology and Criminal Justice" Florida State University.

KI Kaitian. 2003. "A Tribute to Dr.Louis C. Lasagna: 1923-2003." *Drug Information Journal* 37: 353–54.

L Vostry, I Kracikova, B Hofmanova, V Czernekova, T Kott, and J Pribyl. 2011. "Intra-Line and Inter-Line Genetic Diversity in Sire Lines of the Old Kladruber Horse Based on Microsatellite Analysis of DNA." *Czech Journal of Animal Science* 56 (4): 163–75.

LA Seidman, and N Warren. 2001. "Educating the Biotechnology Workforce: Pharmaceutical Regulation in the United States." *Biolink*.

"Law for the Prevention of Offspring with Hereditary Diseases (July 14, 1933). Document 3067-PS, Pp. 880-83". In US Chief Counsel for the Prosecution of Axis Criminality, Nazi Conspiracy and Aggression. Volume 5, Washington, DC: United States Government Printing Office, 1946.

"Louis C. Lasagna Papers (1947-2001)." 2014. River Campus Libraries at University of Rochester: Department of rare books, special collections, and preservation. Accessed May 11.

Louis Lasagna. 1962. *Doctor's Dilemmas*. NY: Harper & Row.

Loving vs. Virginia. 1967. U.S. Supreme Court.

Luebke, David M. 2014. "The Spread of Plague."

Lutz Kaelber. 2012. "Washington: Eugenics: Compulsory Sterilization in 50 American States. Available At:" presented at the Social Science History Association.

Lutz Kaelber. "Oregon: Eugenics: Compulsory Sterilization in 50 American States.

M Davis. 2003. "What Can We Learn by Looking for the First Code of Professional Ethics?" *Theoretical Medicine and Bioethics* 24 (5): 433–54.

M Parrish. *Sacrifice of the Generals: Soviet Senior Officer Losses, 1939-1953; Pp 97-100.* Scarecrow Press, Inc.

Maimonides, Moses. 1204a. *Commentary of the Mishnah: Kitab Al-Siraj (Sefer Ha-Maor, Perush Ha-Mishnah).*

Muslim Philosophy. 1204b. *The Book of the Commandments: Kitab Al-Fara'id (Sefer Ha-Mitzvot).*

Moses Maimonides. 1204c. *The Guide for the Perplexed.* Translated from the original Arabic text by M. Friedlander.

Mary C Gillett. "Lawson's Last Years, 1846-1861." In *The Army Medical Department 1818-1865,* edited by David F. Trask. Office of Medical History - U.S. Army Medical Department.

Office of Medical History - U.S. Army Medical Department. "The Civil War, 1861: Many Problems, Few Solutions." In *The Army Medical Department 1818-1865,* edited by David F. Trask.

Matza, Louis. 2012. "The Sacred Nature of Secular Medicine in the Time of the Black Death". New Brunswick, New Jersey: Rutgers University.

McLaughlin vs. Florida. 1964. U.S. Supreme Court.

Michael Kalish. 2004. "Friedrich Nietzsche's Influence on Hitler's Mein Kampf". UCSB.

MJ Drake, IW Mills, and D Cranston. "The Eugenics Movement. Quoted and from 'The Chequered History of Vasectomy.'" *British Journal of Urology.*

"Modern Oath." 2014. Indian Medical Association.

Molly Billings. "The Influenza Pandemic of 1918."

Moses Maimonides. 1917. "The Oath of Maimonides and The Prayer of Maimonides." *Bulletin of the Johns Hopkins Hospital* 28: 260–61.

N Lakhani. 2011. "From Tragedy to Travesty: Drugs Tested on Survivors of Bhopal." *The Independent*, November 15.

National Geographic's Battle for Midway. 2001. National Geographic Videos.

National Security Council Staff. 1972. "Foreign Relations of the United States, 1969–1976, Volume E–13, Documents on China, 1969–1972, Document 86: MEMORANDUM Memorandum for the President. From: Henry A Kissinger: Your Meetings with Mao". U.S. Department of State: Office of the Historian.

Naval Historical Center. "USS Chesapeake (1800-1813)."

Nazi Conspiracy and Aggression: Opinion and Judgment. Office of United States Chief of Counsel for Prosecution of Axis Criminality. 1949. Washington, DC: U.S. Government Printing Office.

News Medical. 2014. "History of Thalidomide." *News Medical.*

Nora Krug. 2003. "Louis Lasagna, 80, a Doctor and an Expert on Placebos, Dies." *The New York Times*, August 11.

Office of the Chief of Military History, United States Army. "American Military History, Army Historical Series: The War of 1812."

Orent, Wendy. 2012. *Plague: The Mysterious Past and Terrifying Future of the World's Most Dangerous Disease.* Free Pres.

P Brewer. 2007. *The Chronicle of War. A Year-by-Year Account of Conflict from 1854 to the Present Day. P 62.* Carlton Books Ltd.

Pace v. State of Alabama. 1883. U.S. Supreme Court.

"Physician Oaths." 2014. American Association of Physicians and Surgeons: Accessed May 11. www.aapsonline.org/ethics/oaths.htm.

Prager KM. 1987. "Soviet Health Care's Critical Condition." *The Wall Street Journal*, January 29.

Prince vs. Massachusetts. 1944. U.S. Supreme Court.

R Shilkret. 2004. "Mental Retardation in America: A Historical Reader. The History of Disability." Edited by Steven Noll and James W. Trent, Jr. *Bulletin of the History of Medicine. New York: New York University Press* 79 (2): 354–55.

Radomyski, Mateusz. 2011. "Medical Oaths: When Religion and Ethics Collide." *Amsterdam Law Forum* 3 (1): 68–80.

Rebello, L. 2004. "Revised Doctors Oath. Independent Media Center India". Independent Media Center.

Reich WT. 1995. "The Oath of the School of Enjuin." *Encyclopedia of Bioethics*. Revised Edition Vol 5. New York: Simon & Schuster MacMillan.

Reuters. 2014. "Thalidomide Inventors Apologize for Birth Defects, 50 Years Later."

Rev. Claude Hermann Walter Johns. 1910. "The Eleventh Edition of the Encyclopaedia Britannica."

Richard Weikart. 2003. "Progress through Racial Extermination: Social Darwinism, Eugenics, and Pacifism in Germany, 1860-1918." *German Studies Review* 6.

RL Dugdale. 1891. *The Jukes. A Study in Crime, Pauperism, Disease, and Heredity, Also Further Studies of Criminals*. G.P. Putnam's Sons, The Knickerbocker Press.

Roemo Dallaire. 2004. *Shake Hands with the Devil. The Failure of Humanity in Rwanda*. Da Capo Press.

RT Kronenbitter. 2014. "Leon Trotsky, Dupe of the NKVD. How the Soviets Destroyed the Fourth International." *CIA Library – Center for the Study of Intelligence*. Accessed May 11.

S Scheindlin. 2009. "The Problematic Placebo. Reflections: Science in Cultural Context." *Molecular Interventions* 9 (3): 108–13.

SA Pai, and SK Pandya. 2010. "Speaking for Ourselves. A Revised Hippocratic Oath for Indian Medical Students." *The National Medical Journal of India* 23 (6): 360–61.

Sandlow, LJ. 2012. "Oaths, Codes, and Charters in Medicine over the Ages." *Hektoen International – A Journal of Medical Humanities* 3 (3).

Sawyer, RD. 2007. *The TAO of Deception. Unorthodox Warfare in Historic and Modern China. Chapter Sui and T'ang Conflicts, Pp 189 – 211.* Basic Books.

Schat, Marjolein. 1999. "Justinian's Foreign Policy and the Plague: Did Justinian Create the First Pandemic?" *Insects, Disease, and History.*

SH Harris. 1999. "Japanese Medical Atrocities in World War II: Unit 731 Was Not an Isolated Aberration." In Tokyo, Japan.

Shamshad A Khan. 2009. "Japan: CBW. Institute for Defense Studies and Analyses." *CBW Magazine*, October. http://www.idsa.in/cbwmagazine/Japan-CBW_skhan_1009#footnote9_fsmkbhg.

Sipos, Sorin, Mircea Brie, Ioan Horga, Igor Sarov, and Ion Gumenai. 2010 "Imperial Politics in the East and West of the Romanian Space". University of Oradea, Stat University of Moldova.

Skinner v. Oklahoma Ex Rel. Williamson. 1942.

"SS Marriage Order (December 31, 1931). Document 2284-PS [The History, Mission, and Organization of the Schutzstaffeln of the NSDAP, Compiled on the Commission of the Reichsführer-SS by the SS-Standartenführer Gunter d'Alquen, 1939], Pp. 976-77." 1931. In United States Chief Counsel for the Prosecution of Axis Criminality, Nazi Conspiracy and Aggression, Volume IV. Washington, DC: United States Government Printing Office, 1946.

Steven Nadler. "Baruch Spinoza." *Stanford Encyclopedia of Philosophy.* Stanford University. 2001.

TB Heritage. 2014. "Thoroughbred Heritage: Foundation Sires."

Terrence Mallick. 1998. *The Thin Red Line.*

The Library of Congress. "American Memory: Louisiana: European Explorations and the Louisiana Purchase."

The Library of Congress. "Primary Documents in American History – Louisiana Purchase."

The National Archives. "British Transatlantic Slave Trade." https://www.nationalarchives.gov.uk/records/research-guides/slave-trade-slavery.htm.

The National Archives. "Medieval Concept of Human Rights 1215-1500." *The National Archives.*

The Nuremberg Code. 1947. Trials of War Criminals before the Nuremberg Military Tribunals under Control Council Law No. 10, Vol. 2, pp. 181-182. Washington, D.C.: U.S. Government Printing Office, 1949. ohsr.od.nih.gov/guidelines/nuremberg.html.

"The Reich Citizenship Law of September 15, 1935, and the First Regulation to the Reich Citizenship Law of November 14, 1935 Documents 1416-PS and 1417-PS, Pp. 7-10." 2014. In United States Chief Counsel for the Prosecution of Axis Criminality, Nazi Conspiracy and Aggression, Volume IV. Washington, DC: United States Government Printing Office, 1946.

"The Reich Citizenship Law of September 15, 1935, and the First Regulation to the Reich Citizenship Law of November 14, 1935. Documents 1416-PS and 1417-PS, Pp. 7-10." 2014. In United States Chief Counsel for the Prosecution of Axis Criminality, Nazi Conspiracy and Aggression, Volume IV. Washington, DC: United States Government Printing Office, 1946.

Thomas Percival. *Medical Jurisprudence; Or, A Code of Ethics and Institutes Adapted to the Professions of Physic and Surgery (1794).*

"Thomas Percival (1740 – 1804)."*Reynolds Historical Library.*

"Torah Class: Rediscovering the Old Testament. Lesson 1, Introduction to Leviticus Part 1." 2014. *Old Testament Studies.*

Troy Riemer. "How Colonialism Affected the Rwandan Genocide."

U.S. Immigration Act of 1924. 1924.

"U.S. Strategic Bombing Survey. The Effects of the Atomic Bombings of Hiroshima and Nagasaki. Chairman's Office, June 19, 1946." *The Truman Library*. Project Whistlestop.

U.S. Supreme Court. 1927. *Buck v. Bell*. U.S. Supreme Court.

University of Ohio. "Great Britain And The Revolutions of 1848." *Encyclopedia of 1848 Revolutions*.

Vanneste, SF. "The Black Death and the Future of Medicine". Wayne State University. 2010.

Walker, Cameron. "Bubonic Plague Traced to Ancient Egypt." *National Geographic News*. 2004.

Walter Littlefield "Criminal Is a Defective, but Not a Type; Conclusions from Biometrical Study of 3,000 British Convicts Discredit Lombroso's Theory and Minimize the Influence of Environment." *The New York Times*, December 21, 1919.

Washington Revised Code: 1909 c 249 § 35; RRS § 2287, Prevention of Procreation. 1909 c 249 § 35; RRS § 2287.

Wheelis, Mark. "Biological Warfare at the 1346 Siege of Caffa." *Emerg Infect Dis [serial Online]*, September 2002.

William E Seidelman. "Nuremberg Lamentation: The Forgotten Victims of Medical Science." *BMJ*, 313. 1996.

William Ruddick. "Do Doctors Undertreat Pain? Or, The Prayer of Maimonides." *Bioethics* 11 (3/4). 1997.

World Medical Association. "International Code of Medical Ethics". World Medical Association. 1949.

World Medical Association, Geneva. "The Declaration of Geneva." 1948.

Yelena Aronova-Tiuntseva, and Clyde Herreid Freeman. "Hemophilia: 'The Royal Disease'. National Center for Case Study Teaching in Science". University at Buffalo, State University of New York.

Youell, Greg. "The Bible and the Catholic Church." *Bible Research*. 2003.

www.ingramcontent.com/pod-product-compliance
Lightning Source LLC
Chambersburg PA
CBHW051457170526
45166CB00001B/285